THE
DYSPHAGIA
COOKBOOK

THE DYSPHAGIA COOKBOOK

*Great Tasting
and Nutritious Recipes
for People with
Swallowing Difficulties*

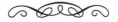

ELAYNE ACHILLES, ED.D

FOREWORD BY TODD LEVINE, M.D.

CUMBERLAND HOUSE
AN IMPRINT OF SOURCEBOOKS, INC.

This book is dedicated to my partner, Jackie. At this time, ALS (Lou Gehrig's disease) has rendered her incapable of eating anything by mouth, so she receives all her food intake through a feeding tube. But as my chief taster, menu adviser, and computer technician, she remains vitally involved in the production of this book. Reviewing the recipes reminds us both of our eating adventures during our relationship and throughout the progress of the disease. Today we continue to prepare dinners for our friends, some of whom experience eating problems. This book is also dedicated to them and to others who are losing the basic vital function of eating. We trust that this book will help them enjoy tasty food that is easy to swallow and to deal with these frustrations in a creative and optimistic manner.

Copyright © 2004 by Elayne Achilles

Published by
Cumberland House Publishing
An Impint of Sourcebooks, Inc.
P.O. Box 4410
Naperville, IL 60567-4410
www.sourcebooks.com

Cover design: Karen Phillips
Text design: Mary Sanford

Library of Congress Cataloging-in-Publication Data
Achilles, Elayne.
  The dysphagia cookbook : great tasting and nutritious recipes for people with swallowing difficulties / Elayne Achilles; foreword by Todd Levine.
     p. cm.
Includes index.
  1. Deglutition disorders—Diet therapy. 2. Cookery (Soft foods) I. Title.
RM221.D4A26 2004
616.3'20654—dc22

                                       2003023856

Printed in the United States of America
RRD 1 0 9 8 7 6 5 4

Contents

Foreword

The ability to eat is one of our basic necessities, but the physical act of swallowing is one of the most complicated acts performed by the nervous system. Swallowing requires the organized actions of brain, nerves, and muscles coordinated with a properly functioning stomach. Further, swallowing necessitates opening the food pipe, or esophagus, while simultaneously closing the airpipe, or trachea, to prevent food from entering the lungs. Pneumonia can develop from food inadvertently entering the trachea.

The complex machinery of swallowing can be easily compromised by many factors. People who suffer from Amyotrophic Lateral Sclerosis (ALS), as well as those who are afflicted with other neurological diseases, may develop difficulty swallowing (dysphagia). In order to grasp why this occurs, it is first necessary to understand the swallowing mechanism and gain some insight into the complexities of the neurological system. Armed with this knowledge, patients of neurological maladies can take steps to moderate the downward spiral of their illnesses.

How the Brain Works

The brain can be viewed as an extremely intricate telecommunications center that starts all physical processes. Every message begins in the brain. Signals to speak, think, move, or feel are transmitted through electrical impulses carried by nerves, which all connect in a complicated pattern similar to telephone wiring. Connections between one nerve and the next allow the signals to be transmitted. In other words, the human body has not yet developed wireless technology.

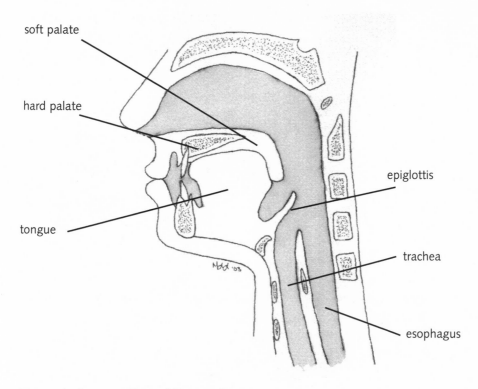

Figure 1: Cross section of the oropharynx.

The initial impulse to move any muscle occurs in the front part of the brain, called the frontal lobe. The messages involved in swallowing then travel down to a part of the brain called the brain stem. The brain stem contains the needed structures to send signals to the muscles to move. These relay stations in the brain stem, called nuclei, act as a type of command and control station. Damage to these nuclei often causes irreversible loss of swallowing function. However, damage to the brain may cause only temporary swallowing problems, which may diminish as the brain develops alternative pathways to reach the nuclei in the brain stem. Once the movement impulses leave the brain stem, they travel on specialized

nerve pathways to reach the muscles. It is the organized contraction of these muscles that actually causes movement. Damage to any of these structures or pathways can cause swallowing problems.

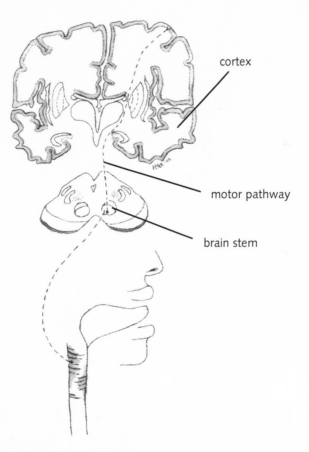

cortex

motor pathway

brain stem

Figure 2: Schematic of the motor pathway to the oropharynx.

AMYOTROPHIC LATERAL SCLEROSIS

ALS, or Lou Gehrig's disease, has afflicted Jackie Boswell, who is my patient and the inspiration for this book. She is an outstanding woman who serves as an example of how to live meaningfully in terrible situations. Lou Gehrig's disease affects 1 in 100,000 people. This ailment may start at any age, in any person, and in any muscle or part of the body. It slowly kills the nerves that make the muscles move. Over the course of two to five years, this disease prevents people from moving their arms, legs, tongue, and breathing muscles. Eventually they are unable to breathe or swallow on their own. At this point they must choose to go on either a breathing machine or a ventilator, or to pass away. Stephen Hawking is a famous example of someone who has lived on a ventilator for many years. However, in my practice, I have seen this as a difficult existence for patients and their families. Despite the slow but incessant progression of muscle death, the mind and thinking remain unaffected. At present there is no effective treatment to stop the decline and eventual death of people affected by ALS.

One of the struggles that face people with ALS is that they are rendered unable to talk or swallow during their illness because the nerves will not tell their muscles to move. Food intake decreases, resulting in increased weakness or even starvation. However, there is hope that through proper nutrition precious time can be added to a patient's life.

While we still do not have an effective treatment for ALS, we know that adequate nutrition throughout the course of their illness can extend patients' lives. This means finding foods in the early stages of the disease that are easy to swallow and packed with nutrition. This book fulfills that need, offering invaluable advice on how to maintain healthy food intake even when suffering from dysphagia. As chewing and swallowing difficulties advance, many patients in my clinic, including Jackie, decide to have a feeding tube placed so they can receive most of their nutrition without having to work so hard to eat. This allows them more energy to enjoy foods they like.

STROKE AND OTHER NEUROLOGIC DISEASES CAUSE DYSPHAGIA AS WELL

Swallowing problems are not solely limited to ALS patients but unfortunately plague many other people who suffer from a variety of neurological problems. Stroke affects 750,000 Americans a year and is the third leading cause of death in the United States. Strokes can occur as a result of blood clots forming in the arteries that supply the brain with blood, or they can occur when a blood vessel in the brain ruptures. The damage caused by a stroke depends entirely on which part of the brain is injured. If the frontal lobes of the brain are damaged or the nuclei in the brain stem are damaged, people will develop dysphagia, or difficulty swallowing. Because swallowing improperly can cause pneumonia, which can prove fatal following a stroke, many doctors do not allow stroke patients to eat until they have been evaluated by a speech pathologist. If a patient's swallowing is damaged by stroke, they may have to use a feeding tube for some time following their stroke. Many patients regain their ability to swallow within six months to a year, but some retain permanent limitations.

There are some cases of treatable types of muscle diseases that may limit one's ability to swallow. Polymyositis and dermatomyositis are autoimmune diseases. This means that the immune system, which is designed to protect our bodies by fighting bacteria and viruses, has gone awry. In these cases the immune system attacks one's own muscles, causing significant muscle weakness. The good news for these patients is that we have many different medications to suppress the immune system, often leading to return of normal muscle function. However, patients must cope with the side effects of taking medications that weaken the ability to fight infections.

Another treatable autoimmune disease called myasthenia gravis frequently causes swallowing problems. In this disease the signal from the nerve to the muscle is interrupted, resulting in muscle that remains healthy but cannot contract because it doesn't receive the proper signals from the nerve. Severely affected patients may have profound swallowing problems requiring feeding tubes until doctors get their disease in remission. When weakness develops to a crisis point patients are often placed in the hospital. Skilled monitoring is important because when swallowing muscles are affected often breathing muscles are affected as well, possibly resulting in death if not treated aggressively.

Some untreatable muscle diseases that may cause swallowing problems include a long list of inherited diseases such as muscular dystrophies. Some cause difficulties from birth or early childhood, while others progress more slowly and create serious problems in adult life. Another untreatable muscle disease called inclusion body myositis is a degenerative disease of the muscle. As patients with this disease age, their muscles start to deteriorate. Patients with inclusion body myositis often develop severe swallowing problems. Since science has not yet advanced to a point where we can treat the cause of these diseases, we must find alternative ways to combat the muscular weakness, such as feeding patients with a feeding tube.

I am proud to have helped Jackie and her partner, Elayne, cope with living with ALS. They are examples of courage and generosity of spirit. My fervent wish is that this cookbook will bring better nutrition to those who are compelled to use it, contributing to a more pleasant today and a longer tomorrow. On the surface the author is writing about food, but in reality she is speaking about human dignity.

TODD D. LEVINE, M.D.,
CLINICAL ASSISTANT PROFESSOR, UNIVERSITY OF ARIZONA,
DIRECTOR OF SAMARITAN ALS CLINIC

Acknowledgments

Susan Brumley, R.D., nutritionist at the ALS Clinic in Phoenix, Arizona, was the first person to suggest writing a cookbook for those with eating difficulties, since there was such a lack of creative solutions in print. Her appreciation of our efforts gave us the confidence that a dysphagia cookbook was needed and possible.

Pamela Mathy, Ph.D., CCC-SLP, Director of Clinical Services at Arizona State University's Speech and Hearing Clinic, supplied the information on general swallowing recommendations and general food considerations that appear in the Introduction. Her individual work with Jackie as well as her many public presentations and writings on dysphagia helped crystallize the principles on which to base the recipes.

Jackie's neurologist, Todd Levine, M.D., Clinical Assistant Professor at the University of Arizona and Director of Samaritan ALS Clinic, graciously wrote the Foreword. He understands eating difficulties on a personal level, since during the writing of this book he experienced a temporary feeding tube placement. He enlisted his wife, Mary Landau-Levine, M.D., Pathologist with Scottsdale Healthcare, to create the sketches for the Foreword that illustrate the swallowing mechanism and neuromuscular pathways. Our deepest appreciation extends to Dr. Levine for inspiring his patients and their caregivers to take proactive measures in their own care.

Many of our friends and relatives contributed recipes or cooking ideas, which have been incorporated into the book. We appreciate the special efforts they devoted to the project and thank them for the good meals and hospitality at their homes.

The staff of the ALS Association, Arizona Chapter, has been a constant source of moral and physical support. Through the Association we have met and received inspiration from patients and caregivers. We have also learned much about courage and commitment from Curt Schilling, star pitcher for the Arizona Diamondbacks and an Honorary Spokesman for the ALSA, and his wife, Shonda, who serves on the board of directors.

Ron Pitkin, president of Cumberland House Publishing, saw the need for this type of book, and editor Mary Sanford paid thoughtful attention to myriad details. I gratefully acknowledge their support.

Introduction

In January of 2001 Jackie, my partner of seventeen years, was diagnosed with Amyotrophic Lateral Sclerosis (ALS), more commonly known as Lou Gehrig's disease. Our lives were changed forever. In Jackie's case the muscle weakness occurred first in her voice and throat, making speech, chewing, and swallowing progressively difficult. Since enjoying and entertaining with great food and wine is one of the staples of our relationship, we challenged ourselves to create new ways to maintain our pleasure in cooking and sharing food. Since the time of that fateful diagnosis, we have encountered many people with chewing and swallowing difficulties who are looking for tasty foods that are easy to chew and swallow. Dieticians and speech pathologists have encouraged our culinary adventures, since there are so few resources for people with dysphagia.

If you or someone you love or care for has difficulties chewing and swallowing, this book is for you. The recipes in this book are focused on the pleasure of eating, something greatly desired when a person's eating capabilities are limited. There are several medical conditions that may cause chewing and swallowing difficulties. Neurological diseases such as ALS, Parkinson's disease, multiple sclerosis, and cerebral palsy can greatly affect one's ability to chew and swallow effectively. These progressive neurological diseases are particularly difficult because the affected person advances through increasing levels of dysphagia (difficulty swallowing), requiring different methods of food preparation. Cancer, particularly esophageal and laryngeal cancer, can also seriously affect the ability to eat. Likewise, many dental problems can cause eating difficulties, if only on a temporary basis. It is assumed that the person using these recipes maintains a fairly reasonable intake of nutrition and hydration from other sources, such as nutritional drinks and supplements or the use of a feeding tube. Although the recipes use nutritious ingredients, they focus on enhancing flavor, presentation, texture, aroma, and color more than simply providing nutritious calories or liquids.

Eating is a social activity. The domestic ritual of eating gives shape and meaning to our lives. Many meals are consumed in a pleasant atmosphere with the company of loved ones and friends in lively conversation. Sustenance is based on a complex of all these considerations. The sounds of clinking silverware and conversation mingled with the aroma of food provide an essential setting for well-being. The primary purpose of the recipes and suggestions found on the following pages serves to heighten this pleasant ritual. Limitations of the mechanics of eating should interfere as little as possible with maintaining the social aspects of eating.

Ease of preparation is also an important consideration for making easy-eating recipes. Many of these meals will be prepared by someone who cares deeply about the person with eating difficulties. Or the person for whom this book is written may be making these recipes under certain physical limitations. Therefore the recipes offer simple alternatives to foster ease of preparation. However, for special occasions, you might want to make the most of the moment and prepare the best. Many of the recipes are suitable as designed for all diners; in some cases, suggestions are made for adapting the family entrée to make it more suitable for the affected individual. Certain processes, such as blending, puréeing, and ricing, are included because frequently many of these techniques are not employed in normal cooking. This is not a comprehensive cookbook. It includes recipes that we particularly like or that are easy to prepare. (We have found that some recipes, like crème brûlée, for example, have complicated steps, such as browning under the broiler or using a torch to get the great caramelized top! Our local restaurant serves a mean crème brûlée, and they are happy to see us, even if we only order dessert and coffee, so we leave that one to the professionals.) We hope these recipes will give readers many more ideas of how to create delicious meals that are easy to chew and swallow.

The Eating Environment

Eating habits change as a person deals with eating problems. It may take much longer to eat than before. Or it may be difficult to hold a conversation while trying to concentrate on chewing and swallowing. The person may eat while sitting in bed, may choke when trying to swallow, or spill food on clothing, table, chair, or floor. Food may get cold before one is able to eat. Other diners may finish their meals well before the person with eating difficulties. Many napkins and aprons will undoubtedly be used, as well as different eating and drinking utensils. All these changes can be frustrating and humiliating to the affected person, while also creating tension among the other diners. People who live and eat together need to change ingrained habits of this important ritual in order to accommodate these problems and avoid adding to the affected person's frustration.

Where once it was considered taboo to watch TV or a video while eating, it may be a relief for all to watch a favorite show (possibly recorded ahead for viewing at meals) to allow the person to eat without having to attempt conversation. Planning for this kind of activity at meals might include setting up a table in front of the TV or moving the TV to the dining area. People who finish eating first should always plan on staying at the table until the slower eater is finished. They can drink another glass of water or coffee, or bring something to the table, such as reading material, to share with the loved one while eating. Likewise, people with eating problems will increase their level of family participation by joining in all meals, if only to eat a very small portion of specially prepared food. It is difficult to fathom the losses a person suffers when his or her food choices become increasingly narrow. Families can benefit from sharing emotional issues relating to these problems. As frustrating as it is for the affected person to watch others eat foods he or she can no longer enjoy, others must eliminate their feelings of guilt about eating those foods in the presence of their loved one or friend, because the social aspect of eating together is crucial.

Tips for Preparation, Serving, and Eating

- If cloths are placed on chairs or tables to take up spills, these should be attractive items that can be cleaned easily every day. Prints hide stains better than solid colors. Wrinkle-free cloth napkins take up little room in the washing machine and add to the pleasure of eating. Look for attractive aprons that wash easily.

- "Downsize" plates, cups, and cutlery to fit smaller serving portions, such as demitasse cups for beverages and custard cups for soup. Pickle forks work well to transfer food comfortably to the mouth.

- Make only one or two recipes at a time. Foods prepared with processors and blenders require more preparation and cleanup time. Being realistic about preparation time will prevent frustration and exhaustion. Homemade items can be paired with prepared foods to provide a complete meal.

- Make the table visually appealing with clean and colorful place mats, napkins, and rings. Use flowers and change centerpieces frequently. Use candlelight or other special lighting and play favorite music to add to the ambiance.

- Make the food visually appealing. Serving a visually appealing plate is as important as having an attractive table. When creating a meal, use a combination of colors and textures placed interestingly on the plate. For example, salmon looks great when placed on a small bed of cooked spinach with a little lemon wedge twisted on top.

- Use colorful combinations. Use mashed sweet potatoes instead of white potatoes for variety. Match with bright green vegetables. Contrast colors of sauces (like the bright orange-yellow color of mango purée) with colors of entrées. Make as much as possible from scratch, because the colors will usually be more vibrant, such as homemade cranberry sauce or applesauce.

- Think texture. Put meringues and cream toppings on custards. Accompany dishes with gravies and other sauces. Pair nuts with vegetables and other foods.

- Enhance flavor and aroma. Use fresh spices when possible. Add sautéed fresh garlic to dishes and fresh citrus rinds and juice when appropriate. Serve meals with wine, which enhances the flavor of food. Add wine or liquor while cooking to enhance flavor. Taste is influenced by aroma, so make simple things from scratch, since they taste so much better and make the kitchen smell good!

- Make room for leftovers. For ease in preparation over a period of time, make large portions of the prepared meal. Then freeze in small single-size freezer bags or containers for easy heating in the microwave. These come in handy when time is short or when providing a serving for the affected person if the family meal is not appropriate.

- Prepare food with love. Since other activities may be curtailed, this is one way of staying connected. It's worth the time and effort.

- Think takeout. A great way to enjoy your favorite restaurant foods is to order takeout, so that you can eat in the privacy and comfort of your own home. You can also grind the food a bit more if necessary and still get the great flavor you crave. Most restaurants go overboard when they know how much you enjoy their food.

General Recommendations for Swallowing

Chewing and swallowing can tax the energy of a person affected by dysphagia. Therefore it is important to eat when rested to help make the process more efficient. Smaller is better. Take smaller bites of food and smaller sips of liquid. "Downsize" plates and cups to match small portions. Smaller utensils make it easier to transfer food to the mouth. Eating smaller meals more frequently is also less fatiguing.

Concentrate on the eating process so that food will be less likely to go down the windpipe and cause choking or aspiration into the lungs. Tilting the chin slightly toward the chest when swallowing also helps prevent food from going into the windpipe. Make sure that each bite or sip has cleared the mouth and throat before taking another bite. Think about swallowing before actually swallowing, bringing the action under voluntary control. It may be necessary to swallow more than once for a bite of food to clear the throat. The use of straws can sometimes help to get liquids neatly into the mouth. Using shorter straws reduces the amount of force needed to suck liquids.

Taking pills can be a chore for anyone, but a person with swallowing difficulties needs to be creative to successfully manage pills. Many vitamins come in powder, liquid, capsule, or tablet form. Tablets can be crushed using a mortar and pestle, or pulverized in a coffee grinder (buy one that you use only for that purpose). Capsules can be taken apart and the contents mixed with thick liquids (check with a pharmacist first about taking time-release capsules in this manner). When filling a prescription, ask the pharmacist for choices of types. If required, some common medications, such as aspirin, even come in suppository form. Many people tilt their heads back to take a pill, but contrary to popular belief, this position can be dangerous, as liquids are more likely to go down the airway. Although it feels counterintuitive, try tilting the head slightly forward with liquid and pill in the mouth. The pill floats to the back of the throat, making swallowing easier. There is no need to position the pill on the back of the tongue with the head-tilt method.

GENERAL FOOD CONSIDERATIONS FOR SWALLOWING

Foods that hold together well in the mouth are easier to chew and swallow. Mashed potatoes, for example, form a mass (or bolus) and are easier to manage. Rice kernels, on the other hand, have a tendency to separate and are difficult to control in the mouth. Even with rice pudding, the custard slides down, leaving the individual rice kernels in the mouth. Ground beef is another food that doesn't easily form a bolus, probably because the inexpensive cuts used for grinding contain gristle. However, filet mignon grinds and binds beautifully. Another option in many recipes that call for ground beef is to substitute eggplant.

Contrary to intuition, thicker, not thinner, liquids are easier to control in the mouth and swallow. Thin liquids have a tendency to seep through weakened lip muscles that cannot make a tight seal. Also, when the epiglottis (the flap of cartilage that covers the opening at the top of the windpipe during swallowing) cannot make a tight seal, thin liquids seep through quickly and cause choking. Thicker liquids, such as milk shakes and smoothies, have more texture and don't spread out around the mouth.

Food Consistency Levels

Although it is difficult to classify foods into definite categories of consistency, the recipes in this book are marked with symbols to suggest general levels of food consistency. With progressive disorders, patients will have to continuously adapt to food that requires more processing to allow for safe swallowing. Look for the following symbols:

S Soft—Foods that have not been prepared with a food processor or blender, but can be chewed easily, such as well-cooked vegetables, thinly sliced luncheon meats, scrambled eggs, etc.

G Grind/Shred/Slice—Foods that have been prepared with the grinding, shredding, or slicing blades of a food processor, such as coleslaw, ham, nuts, etc.

P Purée—Foods that have been prepared in a blender, or have enough liquid to be puréed in the processor or forced through a ricer, food mill, or strainer. Note: Foods that have been prepared by pressing through a food mill or a ricer have a consistency somewhere between ground and puréed. Food maintains more integrity of consistency when using these kitchen tools instead of a blender, because food cellulose remains intact and therefore does not become mushy. When possible, use a food mill or ricer instead of a mixer, blender, or processor for better texture.

MUST-HAVE KITCHEN ITEMS: TOOLS OF THE TRADE

Food processor—Essential. You'll want to leave it out on the counter within easy reach. The seven-cup size is probably big enough for most recipes. No fancy attachments are needed, but the motor should be good. (Cuisinart does make a mini-processor for small jobs, but its motor is noisy and not as effective. However, it can be handy to take on vacations or to friends' houses when invited for meals.) Get friendly with your processor, because you will use it constantly. Check the instruction book for details, but here are some basics to learn. (By the way, don't use the processor for mashed potatoes, they turn to glue.)

- *Chopping and puréeing*—Use the metal blade. Use no more than 2 cups of food at a time. Pulse at a rate of 1 second on, 1 second off until food is coarsely chopped. Then press the ON switch and run continuously until the food is chopped as finely as you want. Check frequently to avoid chopping too finely. Use a spatula to scrape down any pieces that stick to the side of the work bowl. It is not necessary to add liquid when preparing foods in a processor.
- *Slicing and shredding*—Use the slicing or shredding disk. Slice food to fit into the feed tube on the lid. Insert the pusher, pushing the food down with one hand and holding the switch down with the other hand until the food is sliced or shredded.
- *Mixing*—Use the plastic blade. Good for mixing batters.

Blender—Get the kind with an easy screw-off base, for easy cleaning and assembling and so fingers don't get punctured on the blade.

The blender does not mix food, it cuts food, but it's not as controlled as a processor. It does a good job on puréed foods, such as fruit smoothies and soups. It's also good for making small portions of crushed ice and small portions of Hollandaise sauce. The processor usually works better for meat, cheese, chopped vegetables, and so on. Place liquid in the blender first before adding solid foods.

Mixer—The blades of a mixer don't cut, they whip air into food. Use for meringues, whipped cream, cake mixes, and so on.

Food mill—A food mill is a metal bowl with holes in the base that hooks over most kitchen bowls. It has a handle in the center with a flat blade attached that forces food through the holes when the handle is turned. This item makes life easy for making applesauce or removing hulls and skins from foods such as apples, tomatoes, corn, or beans. Hulls and skins are left behind. A food mill is essential if small pieces cause choking (which is why it's often used to make homemade baby food). Even puréed foods leave small pieces. Also, the food mill doesn't destroy the fiber makeup of food. While processing food, turn the handle in the opposite direction every now and then to loosen food from the screen.

Ricer—This tool is similar to a garlic press, only larger, and a preferred substitute for mashing with a mixer. Potatoes don't get gooey when using a ricer as they do when processing or mixing. Use for mashed potatoes, squash, and similar dishes.

Slow cooker (also known as a crock pot)—This is a great tool for cooking fork-tender roasts and for serving and keeping soup hot at a party.

High-temperature rubber spatula—Can be used for cooking as well as scraping bowls. Found in most kitchen supply stores.

Small ovenproof ramekins—Use for making individual custards, soufflés, etc. Also good for serving small portions of soup or cereal.

Ovenproof containers—Look for sets with glass and plastic covers that can be used for cooking, refrigerator and freezer storage, and reheating. Really saves on cleanup.

Microwave-safe mixing bowls—Processed food loses heat quickly, so make double use of mixing bowls by using plastic or glass microwave-safe bowls to reheat prepared food for serving. Also double as serving and storage bowls.

Garlic press and garlic—There is no adequate substitute for fresh garlic. Garlic bulbs keep well unrefrigerated in a ventilated jar made for that purpose. Peel by pressing down on the garlic clove with the flat side of a large knife. The peel comes off easily and the clove can then be placed in the garlic press.

Mortar and pestle—A small bowl and mallet to pulverize tablets into a powder. Mix powder with other foods for ease in taking pills. Also look for pills in capsule form. Capsules can be opened and the powder mixed with food. Some medication comes in liquid form and can be mixed with food. Mortars and pestles can be found in kitchen supply stores or specialty shops.

Coffee grinder—Works even better than a mortar and pestle for grinding pills. Use a small brush to remove all powder from the machine.

Fresh herbs—Essential for tasty food. Keep flowerpots filled with your favorite herbs on the windowsill, or, if you live in a warm climate, keep an herb garden outside. Rosemary, basil, and parsley are essential. Chives, thyme, sage, and tarragon are good too.

PANTRY AND REFRIGERATOR SUPPLIES

Yoplait Nouriche—A thick blend of fruits and yogurt. Thicker than Tropicana Smoothies. Find in the dairy case of the grocery store. Good for taking pills.

Glen Oaks Tropical Fruit Drink—Drinkable yogurt and puréed fruits. About as thick as Nouriche. Great taste.

Hansen's Smoothies—In a can. Many flavors. Pineapple coconut is great with rum. Thicker than juice, but not as thick as Nouriche.

Kern's brand nectars and Jumex brand nectars—In a can. Various flavors. Thicker than juice. Look for Looza brand nectars from Belgium in a tall jar. A taste test revealed Looza was better than the others. Great thick liquid for taking pills.

Six-ounce cans of juices, such as pineapple, prune, and apple—Good for making smoothies and for traveling.

Dannon La Crème—An incredibly creamy and mild yogurt that comes in 4-ounce sizes. The smaller serving portion is more appealing and makes for less contamination of leftovers. Look for 4-ounce yogurts that are made with whole milk, which makes them rich and creamy.

Yoplait Whips—Yogurt with a light and fluffy texture.

Individual snack packs of applesauce, puddings, etc.—Usually do not need refrigeration and are a convenient size to slip into a bag or glove compartment of the car. Great to take on outings. Mott's mixed berry Fruitsations has a great color.

Del Monte Mango—In extra light syrup. Chunks of mango in a quart jar. Great substitute for fresh mango and saves preparation time. Works well in yogurt smoothies. Use the light syrup as part of the liquid.

Commercially prepared flan mix—This Spanish-style dessert or breakfast custard can be found in the international section of the grocery store. It's a great substitute for homemade.

Junket Rennet Tablets or Custard Mix—Makes a delicate rennet custard or thick milk drink. Rennet is a natural substance that coagulates milk.

Matzo ball soup mix—Can be found in the Kosher food section of the grocery store. Comes in a variety of packaging. Matzo balls are made from matzo meal, which is a finely ground wheat. It makes an easy-to-eat dumpling that tastes great in chicken broth.

Potato starch—Found in the Kosher food section of the grocery store. Similar to instant mashed potatoes but without seasonings. Can be used as a thickener for almost any food.

Hummus (spread made with chickpeas), babaganouj (spread of roasted eggplant with tahini, a sesame seed paste), and tzatziki (cucumber yogurt sauce)—All can be found in most grocery stores and taste great. It's not worth the effort to make these from scratch. Usually eaten as a dip with pita bread.

Mini whole wheat pitas—To keep fresh, use zippered snack bags to freeze small amounts. To thaw, wrap a few pitas in a paper towel and warm in the microwave for 15 seconds on high power.

Cocktail breads—Very small loaves that are usually found in the deli. Easier to manage than regular-size slices and have almost no crust. The loaf can be kept fresh by dividing into small portions and freezing in zippered bags.

Falafel mix (in a box)—Falafel patties are made with ground chickpeas. Any of the three spreads above make a great topping for falafel.

Tabbouleh mix (in a box)—Tabbouleh is made with bulgur wheat and mixed with lots of parsley, mint, and fresh tomatoes. Forms a bolus (mass) in the mouth more easily than rice.

Stouffer's Vegetable Lasagna—In the frozen foods section of the grocery store. Comes in twelve-serving size and smaller serving sizes. Works well for company or fast meals when you don't want to or can't cook.

Bear Creek Broccoli Cheese Soup—Comes in packets of powder in the soup section of the grocery store. Nice and thick for easy swallowing. Just add liquid to the amount desired and save the remainder for future use. Can be used as a base for sauces too.

Liverwurst—Makes a great luncheon spread.

Arrowroot—A delicate starch thickener used in place of cornstarch. Find in the spice section of the grocery store. Sauces thickened with arrowroot have a more transparent and natural appearance. Great for thickening fruit sauces (see Poached Pears, p. 134) and Asian sauces. In any recipe that calls for cornstarch, substitute equal amounts of arrowroot. Maximum thickening is reached before boiling occurs.

Unflavored gelatin—Thickens almost anything (see Bloody Mary Aspic, p. 150).

Refried beans—When puréed, they make a nice soup thickener.

Edamame (Ed-ah-MAH-may)—These blanched, shelled soybeans are loaded with protein and can be found in the frozen vegetable section of most grocery stores. They are easier to eat when combined with puréed vegetables, such as sweet potatoes or squash, and also provide added texture to puréed vegetables.

Heaven's Delight tapioca pudding—Find at Costco. This is so good, there's no need to make from scratch.

Oyster crackers—Small enough to put in mouth whole. Let soften in soups (like oyster stew) for easy eating.

Small macaroni shells—Known as conchigliette and found in the pasta section of the grocery store. Because of their small size they are easier to place in the mouth and chew. They are great for macaroni and tuna salad.

Safeway frozen shepherd's pie—Soft and easy to chew and swallow. Beef and mashed potatoes make a hearty meal.

Baker's whipping cream—Contains sugar and vanilla, so it's ready to whip with a mixer for dessert toppings. Also, the cream makes a thick base for sweet alcoholic drinks, or a creamer for coffee.

Confectioners' sugar—Use in place of granulated sugar for quick-dissolving recipes, such as uncooked fruit sauces.

Williams-Sonoma Butternut Squash Purée—Works well as a thickener in soups and sauces. Also can be added to dishes that are too spicy for sensitive palates.

Crème fraîche—Use in place of whipping cream. It's lighter than sour cream, but thick. A dollop of cold crème fraîche on puréed soups provides a nice contrast in color and temperature. Also tastes great on fruits and desserts (see p. 114).

Chicken broth—Comes in 1-cup, 2-cup, and quart-size containers. Keep all sizes on hand for different needs. Comes in handy for thinning foods that are too thick.

Idahoan Instant Mashed Potatoes—Come in 4-ounce packets and large box in several flavors. Just add the packet to boiling water for delicious mashed potatoes. Potato flakes can also be poured directly into soups and sauces as an instant thickener.

Simply Thick—A commercial thickening gel you can't taste. Made with xanthan gum. Just shake, stir, or mix the contents of one packet into the liquid to be thickened. Can be heated. Phagi-Gel Technologies, St. Louis, MO 63011, 800-205-7115, www.simplythick.com. Comes in two consistencies: honey and nectar.

Ham steak—Grinds well in the processor and mixes with cream sauces and soups for a more hearty dish.

Grated Parmesan cheese—Keep on hand for sprinkling on many dishes to provide added protein.

TRAVELING AND EATING OUT

More thought has to be put into having appropriate foods while traveling and eating out when food choices are limited. For traveling in the car, keep a small cooler in the trunk or back seat and have a few small ice packs in the freezer ready for travel. Keep a collection of plastic cutlery, napkins, straws, cups, and possibly an apron for eating on the go. A roll of paper towels comes in handy when traveling in the car. Four-ounce yogurt cups and yogurt drinks are good to pack, because they are thick and more nourishing than milk shakes and puddings found at fast-food restaurants and small enough to eat at one sitting. Take or buy drinks on the road that have twist-off caps, so that small amounts may be consumed and the rest kept in the cooler for future use. Cans of nectars are thicker than soft drinks and easier to control in the mouth. Packs of applesauce and other puddings that don't require refrigeration are good to keep in the glove compartment. Homemade soups that you freeze in small containers work well as ice packs for the cooler and also provide a meal that can be heated quickly in the microwave upon arrival at your destination. Make hotel reservations contingent on the availability of microwaves and small refrigerators in the room. You may want to consider traveling with a mini food processor to prepare foods you enjoy.

If you're lucky enough to find yourself traveling on a ship, consider selecting a cruise that accommodates different styles of dining. Some cruises have only one seating option that places diners at large tables for every meal at fixed times. More cruises now offer flexible restaurant hours and small tables. In this eating environment, you may choose to eat alone or with others and take as much time as you want to eat. This allows the person with eating difficulties to enjoy food without feeling rushed or observed. On cruises, waiters depend on tips from their customers and will go overboard (not quite) to provide food you can enjoy.

Eating in restaurants is a time-honored social activity. Some people with eating difficulties blanch at the idea of finding edible foods on the menu, let alone eating under the gaze of others. Reading the suggestions below should help you feel more confident about food choices in restaurant dining. Remember also that most waiters and chefs will go to considerable effort to serve food according to your needs. There is no law that mandates everyone at the table order an entrée, so ask for an extra plate to share food or order soup or an appetizer instead of an entrée. There is also no law that mandates eating dessert at the end of the meal, so diners should feel comfortable ordering crème brûlée while others eat their entrée. Life is too short to worry about other people's reactions to your eating habits, but if this is a problem, find a table more protected from the view of others. Making the effort to eat out can be a rewarding experience for everyone. However, if you prefer to eat your favorite restaurant food in the privacy of your own home, order takeout!

Below is a basic list of ideas for easy-eating food choices in restaurants:

- At the mall: Orange Julius; juice bars for smoothies; donut shop (pieces of donut can be dunked in coffee and retrieved with a fork or spoon); crush crackers in soup to thicken liquid.
- Mexican restaurant: refried beans with cheese; flan; corn pudding; guacamole; frittata.
- Seafood restaurant: clam or oyster chowder with oyster crackers crushed in; any broiled flaky fish (avoid fried because the crust is hard to swallow); salmon is always good and can be found on most menus.
- Chinese restaurant: egg drop soup (this is thick and does not have as many pieces of food as you might find in hot and sour soup); bean curd (tofu) dishes; eggplant dishes; almond cookie dipped in hot tea.
- Middle Eastern: hummus; babaganouj; tzatziki; falafel; tabbouleh.
- Thai: potato curry in coconut milk (mash the potatoes with a fork and mix into the sauce).

- Italian food: non-meat raviolis (cheese or squash) with alfredo sauce.
- East Indian food: spinach dishes; dahl (lentil-based dishes); raita (yogurt dish with mint and spices); chutney (fruit relish).
- French food: lobster or crab bisques; crème brûlée; crêpes; quiche; vichyssoise; potatoes au gratin.
- Japanese food: miso soup.
- General suggestions: Ask chefs to make something you can eat. They will process foods, such as salad, or purée just about any dish you would like to taste. When friends invite you over for dinner, explain ahead of time any eating issues. Tell them you can bring most of your own food, such as a blended salad. If they ask what you can eat, suggest something simple like a small piece of salmon, or a soft cake dessert.

I

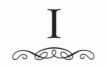

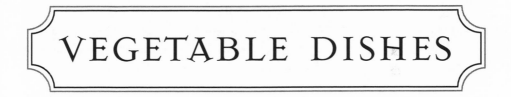

VEGETABLE DISHES

LATKES: POTATO PANCAKES

INGREDIENTS

- 2 large potatoes, peeled
- 1 small onion, peeled
- 2 eggs
- 3 tablespoons milk
- 2 tablespoons melted butter
- ¼ cup flour
  Salt and pepper to taste

PREPARATION

Cut the potatoes and onion to fit the feed tube of the processor, using the shredding disk to grate both. Place the grated potatoes and onion in water as you work to prevent discoloration. Drain the potatoes and onion, squeezing out the excess water by wrapping tightly in a towel. Place in a mixing bowl and set aside. Remove the shredder disk and insert the plastic blade. Add the eggs, milk, and melted butter, and blend. Then add the flour, salt, and pepper, and process until smooth. Pour over the potatoes and onions and stir.

Preheat the griddle to 350°. Drop the potato mixture by large spoonfuls onto the griddle. (Butter the griddle just before frying the pancakes, and re-butter for each batch.) Cook for 4 minutes, then turn and cook for 3 minutes, or until golden brown. Serve with dollops of sour cream and/or applesauce (homemade is really good, see p. 128). Leftover pancakes may be frozen between sheets of waxed paper and reheated in a toaster oven or microwave. Serves 6.

ORZO

Orzo is pasta in the shape of rice. Because orzo forms a bolus (or mass) in the mouth more easily than rice, it makes a good rice substitute. It can be found in the pasta section of most grocery stores in a small box.

INGREDIENTS

3 cups chicken, vegetable, or beef broth

1 cup dry orzo

PREPARATION

In a saucepan heat the broth to boiling. Add the orzo, reduce the heat to simmer, and cook, covered, until the orzo is tender, about 12 minutes. For more interest, mix with sautéed onion, mushrooms, and/or red pepper. Leftovers can be added to canned soups. Serves 4 to 6.

2 pounds boiling potatoes (such as Yellow Finn or Fingerling), peeled

1 celery root, about 1 pound, peeled

Salt to taste

5 tablespoons butter

Minced garlic (optional)

½ cup milk or cream

POTATO AND CELERY ROOT PURÉE

PREPARATION

Cut the potatoes and celery root into pieces. In a saucepan cover the vegetables with water, add the salt, and boil until tender, about 15 minutes. Pass through a food mill or ricer. Add the butter, and add garlic if desired. In a small saucepan warm the milk or cream and stir into the mixture. Serves 4 to 6.

SPICY POTATOES

PREPARATION

In a skillet heat the olive oil and cook the leeks, ginger, garlic, and salt for a few minutes until the leeks are soft. Add the milk and simmer for a few more minutes. Add the pepper, coriander, turmeric, cumin, and peas (with liquid), and simmer for a few more minutes. Add the mixture to the riced potatoes and tofu and mix gently. Goes well with fish. Serves 6.

INGREDIENTS

1	teaspoon olive oil
½	cup minced leeks
2	teaspoons minced fresh ginger
1	small clove garlic, minced
½	teaspoon salt
½	cup milk or half and half
⅛	teaspoon pepper
½	teaspoon ground coriander
⅛	teaspoon turmeric
¼	teaspoon ground cumin
½	cup frozen peas, cooked
2	large potatoes, peeled, boiled, and passed through a ricer
½	cup silken tofu (optional), passed through a ricer

SCALLOPED POTATOES

INGREDIENTS

3 tablespoons butter

¼ onion, minced

3 tablespoons all-purpose flour

2 cups milk

Salt and pepper to taste

½ cup grated Cheddar cheese (optional)

3 large potatoes, peeled and sliced in processor

Ham steak, ground (optional)

PREPARATION

In a saucepan heat the butter and sauté the onion. Add the flour and stir constantly over medium heat for 2 minutes. Remove from the heat. Add the milk slowly, stirring with a whisk. Return to the heat, whisking constantly, until thickened. Add salt and pepper. If desired, add the Cheddar cheese to the sauce.

Preheat the oven to 350°. Layer the potatoes and sauce in an ovenproof casserole with a lid. Cover and bake for about 1 hour. Uncover and continue baking until the top is slightly brown and the potatoes are very tender. If desired, ham steak pulsed a few times in the processor can be mixed into the sauce for a more hearty dish. Serves 6.

MICROWAVE SCALLOPED POTATOES

PREPARATION

In a 2-quart microwave casserole with a lid, melt the butter on high for about 30 seconds (watch carefully so it doesn't boil). Blend in the flour, salt, and pepper. Gradually stir in the milk with a wire whisk and microwave on high for about 8 to 10 minutes, stirring with the whisk every 3 minutes. Mix the shredded potatoes and onion into the casserole. Cover and microwave on high for about 17 to 19 minutes, stirring with a spoon after 10 minutes. Remove from the microwave, sprinkle the Cheddar cheese on top, cover, and let stand for 5 minutes before serving. Serves 4 to 6.

INGREDIENTS

3   tablespoons butter

2   tablespoons all-purpose flour

1   teaspoon salt

¼   teaspoon pepper

2   cups milk

3   medium potatoes, peeled and shredded in processor, using shredding blade

2   tablespoons minced onion

½   cup grated Cheddar cheese

PESTO MASHED POTATOES

INGREDIENTS

2 pounds boiling potatoes, boiled and cut into pieces, or 6 servings instant mashed potatoes

¼ cup homemade pesto sauce (see p. 118) or commercially prepared pesto sauce (more or less according to taste)

PREPARATION

In a saucepan boil the potatoes until tender (or prepare the mashed potatoes according to package directions). Drain the potatoes and press through a ricer into a bowl. Mix in the Pesto Sauce. These potatoes are good served with white fish, because their delicate green color contrasts nicely. Serves 6.

RICED SWEET POTATOES OR YAMS

PREPARATION

Peel and cut the potatoes into chunks, cover with water, and boil until very tender. Press through a ricer (or mash) in a bowl with your choice of butter, sour cream, or cream cheese (or all three), and salt and pepper. You might want to add bourbon, crushed pineapple, or orange juice and grated orange rind to add more interest.

CLAUDIA'S SOUTHWESTERN CANDIED YAMS

INGREDIENTS

- 2 pounds yams
- ⅓ cup red jalapeño jelly
- ⅓ cup finely chopped cilantro
- 2 tablespoons lime juice
- 2 tablespoons tequila

PREPARATION

Peel and cut the yams into chunks. Place in a saucepan, cover with water, and boil until very tender. Press through a ricer. Add the red jalapeño jelly, cilantro, lime juice, and tequila, and serve hot. Goes well with poultry and stuffing. Serves 6.

CARROT AND RUTABAGA PURÉE

INGREDIENTS

1 rutabaga, peeled and chopped into small cubes

3 medium-size carrots, peeled and sliced

3 tablespoons butter

3 tablespoons sour cream

Salt and pepper to taste

PREPARATION

In a saucepan cover the rutabaga and carrots in water, and bring to a boil. Reduce the heat and simmer until very tender, about 25 minutes. Rutabaga takes longer to cook than carrots. Drain, and pass the vegetables through a ricer into a serving bowl. Mix in the butter, sour cream, salt, and pepper. Reheat before serving. Serves 6.

ACORN SQUASH PURÉE

1 acorn squash
2 tablespoons butter
2 tablespoons brown sugar
 Salt and pepper to taste
 Dash nutmeg
1 egg, beaten

PREPARATION

Cut the acorn squash in half lengthwise. Scoop out the seeds and stringy flesh. Place cut side down on a glass baking dish. Cover with plastic wrap, turning one corner up to let the steam escape. Microwave on high until very tender, about 10 minutes. Scoop out the flesh and discard the skins. Press the flesh through a ricer or purée in a food processor. Add the butter, brown sugar, salt, pepper, and nutmeg. *Note:* For a more fluffy dish with added protein, add a beaten egg and bake in a casserole dish in a 350° oven for 30 minutes. *Variation:* You can also make this dish using a combination of acorn squash and turnips instead of just squash. Serves 3 to 4.

POLENTA (CORNMEAL) WITH CHEESE

INGREDIENTS

1½ teaspoons salt

2 cups polenta (cornmeal flour)

4 tablespoons butter

1½ cups grated fontina cheese

PREPARATION

In a large saucepan bring 6 to 8 cups of water to a boil. Add the salt and polenta in a steady stream, whisking constantly to avoid lumps. Reduce the heat and cook for about 30 minutes, stirring frequently. Add a little boiling water while cooking if the mixture gets too thick. Remove from the heat and stir in the butter and cheese. Serving suggestion: Using the back of a spoon, make a depression in a portion of polenta and fill with hot creamed vegetables or meats. Serves 6.

SAUTÉED SPINACH

INGREDIENTS

1 tablespoon olive oil

Fresh garlic (minced)

1 1-pound bag baby spinach

2 teaspoons lemon juice

Salt and pepper to taste

Fresh coriander, minced (optional)

PREPARATION

Heat a large saucepan or wok and add the oil. When the oil is hot, add the garlic and stir-fry for about 30 seconds. Add the spinach and toss until the spinach wilts, about 1 minute. Add the lemon juice, salt, and pepper while tossing. Can be used as a bed for fish, such as salmon or halibut. Just before serving, mix in the coriander. Serves 3 to 4.

PENNSYLVANIA DUTCH SPINACH

PREPARATION

In a saucepan add the flour to the drippings and blend. Add the hot water and cook over low heat until thick, stirring constantly. Add the sugar, vinegar, salt, and pepper. Pour over the spinach and stir until wilted. Serves 4.

INGREDIENTS

Drippings from 4 slices bacon

3 tablespoons all-purpose flour

1½ cups hot water, milk, or combination

2 tablespoons sugar

1 tablespoon vinegar

Salt and pepper to taste

3 cups chopped raw spinach

INGREDIENTS

FRIED SPINACH AND BROCCOLI PURÉE

- 1 cup water
- 1 10-ounce bag washed spinach
- ½ pound fresh broccoli, including tender part of stalks, chopped
- 3 tablespoons butter
- 1 tablespoon fresh gingerroot, peeled and finely chopped
- ½ cup finely chopped onions
- ¼ teaspoon ground cumin
- ¼ teaspoon turmeric
- ½ teaspoon ground coriander
- ½ teaspoon curry powder (optional)
- 1 teaspoon salt (optional)

PREPARATION

In a processor pulse ½ cup water and the spinach until puréed. Transfer to a bowl. Pulse ½ cup water and the broccoli in the processor until puréed, then stir into the puréed spinach. In a heavy skillet melt the butter and sauté the ginger for 1 minute on moderate heat, then add the onions and sauté until the onions are soft. Add the cumin, turmeric, coriander, and curry, frying for a few minutes until well mixed. Stir in the spinach-broccoli mixture a little at a time and fry for 5 minutes. Reduce the heat and simmer, uncovered, for about 15 minutes, until most of the liquid is evaporated. Add the salt if desired. Serves 8.

CREAMED CABBAGE, BROCCOLI, OR CAULIFLOWER

PREPARATION

In the processor slice or grate the cabbage and cook in a microwave-safe dish with a cover (add a few tablespoons water) until very tender, about 6 minutes. Pour the sauce over the cabbage. Add ground almonds if desired. Serves 4.

INGREDIENTS

4 cups cabbage, broccoli, or cauliflower, cut into pieces

1 recipe Basic White Sauce (see p. 110)

Ground almonds, if tolerated

- 1 eggplant
- 2 tablespoons olive oil
- 2 cloves fresh garlic, minced
- 2 tablespoons white wine
- ¼ cup pine nuts, ground in a processor
- Lemon juice to taste
- Grated Parmesan cheese

SAUTÉED EGGPLANT AND PINE NUTS

This makes a great substitute for meat.

PREPARATION

Peel the eggplant and cut into tiny cubes. In a skillet heat the oil and sauté the garlic for about 30 seconds. Add the eggplant and stir to coat. Reduce the heat, add the wine, cover, and cook until the eggplant is soft, about 15 minutes. Add the pine nuts and lemon juice before serving. Eggplant prepared in this fashion makes a wonderful addition when mixed into fresh or prepared pasta sauces and served over very fine egg noodles. Sprinkle a little grated Parmesan cheese on top. Serves 6.

VARIATION: EASY EGGPLANT RATATOUILLE

Preparing ratatouille involves layering eggplant slices, tomatoes, onions, and green pepper. This recipe gives the same flavor without the work.

PREPARATION

Follow the directions for Sautéed Eggplant and Pine Nuts, but after sautéeing the garlic, sauté the onion, green pepper, and tomato. Then add the eggplant and proceed as directed. Add some fresh mint leaves for garnish. *Hint:* Eggplant absorbs oil and will seem very dry when sautéeing. To prevent using too much oil, add a little white wine if the eggplant seems dry. Serves 6.

INGREDIENTS

1   recipe Sautéed Eggplant and Pine Nuts

1   small onion, grated in processor

1   green pepper, grated in processor

1   fresh tomato, skinned and sliced

Fresh mint leaves (optional)

BRAISED RED CABBAGE

INGREDIENTS

- 1 small head red cabbage
- 1 onion
- 1 apple
- ¼ cup sugar
- 1 teaspoon salt
- 1 cup red wine vinegar
- ¼ cup butter
- ½ cup red jelly (jalapeño type optional)
- ¼ cup hot water
- ¼ teaspoon cloves
- ¼ teaspoon cinnamon

PREPARATION

Using the shredding blade of the processor, shred the cabbage, onion, and apple separately. Marinate the cabbage in sugar, salt, and vinegar for 15 minutes. In a saucepan melt the butter and sauté the onion and apple until tender. Add the cabbage mixture and boil. Add the jelly, hot water, cloves, and cinnamon. Cover and simmer for 1 hour. Serve hot as an accompaniment to pulled pork or Little Ham Loaves (see p. 40). Serves 8.

SAUERKRAUT AND APPLES S

PREPARATION

Sometimes tart food can cause choking. To mitigate
the sour taste, add one grated apple and a little
beer to sauerkraut while cooking.

INGREDIENTS

CORN CHILE CUSTARD

2 cups fresh cooked yellow corn kernels (or about 1½ cans whole kernel corn, drained)

1 cup heavy cream

2 eggs

3 egg yolks (Use the reserved egg whites for meringue or to add to scrambled eggs for more protein.)

1 7-ounce can mild diced roasted green chiles (found in Mexican food section of grocery store)

Salt and pepper to taste

Pinch nutmeg

1 teaspoon chili powder

PREPARATION

Preheat the oven to 325°. Grease 7 or 8 ovenproof 5-ounce ramekins or Pyrex custard cups. In a blender combine the corn, cream, eggs, egg yolks, and chiles, and purée until smooth. Strain through a sieve or pass through a food mill. Season with salt, pepper, nutmeg, and chili powder. Pour into the prepared ramekins or custard cups and bake for 25 minutes. Cool and remove from the molds. Goes nicely with a more spicy dish like chicken enchilada soup. Serves 7 to 8.

SPINACH LASAGNE

PREPARATION

Preheat the oven to 350°. In a large bowl mix together the ricotta cheese, Parmesan cheese, parsley, eggs, salt, and pepper. In a 9 x 13-inch pan spoon a layer of sauce to cover the bottom. Press in a layer of noodles to cover. Then spoon half of the ricotta mixture evenly over the noodles and spread a layer of spinach leaves over the ricotta. Layer ½ pound of mozzarella slices evenly over the ricotta. Repeat the layers, adding a layer of noodles and sauce on top. Bake for 45 minutes. Place a cookie sheet on the rack below to catch drips. Serves a crowd, or leftovers can be cut into squares and frozen in zippered bags.

INGREDIENTS

3 cups ricotta cheese

½ cup fresh grated Parmesan cheese

2 tablespoons minced fresh parsley

2 eggs, beaten

2 teaspoons salt (less if using salty tomato sauce)

¼ teaspoon pepper

Your favorite tomato sauce; if using meat sauce, blend first if necessary

Lasagne noodles, uncooked

Fresh spinach leaves (or Swiss chard), washed and stems removed

1 pound mozzarella cheese, sliced thin

PASTA Y FAGIOLI (PASTA AND BEANS)

INGREDIENTS

1¼ cups little white beans or 3 cans undrained cannellini beans
1 vegetable bouillon cube
2 bay leaves
2 to 3 fresh garlic cloves, minced
1 tablespoon olive oil
3 carrots, processed with the shredding blade
2 celery stalks, processed
1 large onion, processed
 Fresh ground pepper
1 tablespoon minced fresh oregano
2 tablespoons minced fresh basil
1 tablespoon minced fresh marjoram
½ cup white wine, not sweet
1 14-ounce can peeled tomatoes
1 cup small shell macaroni or similar small pasta
 Dash Tabasco sauce
 Juice of ½ lemon
 Fresh grated Parmesan cheese to taste
 Minced parsley for garnish

PREPARATION

If using canned beans, place them in a kettle with their liquid. Otherwise, place the beans in a kettle with 6 cups of water for 8 hours.

In the kettle with the beans and water add the bouillon, bay leaves, and garlic. Simmer for about 1 hour 30 minutes. Discard the bay leaves. In a large skillet heat the olive oil and sauté the carrots, celery, and onion. Add the fresh pepper, herbs, wine, and tomatoes, cover, and cook for 10 minutes. In a large saucepan cook the macaroni in boiling salted water until tender. In a large serving bowl combine the beans, veggies, and pasta. Add Tabasco sauce and lemon juice to taste. To serve, sprinkle Parmesan cheese and parsley on top. Tastes even better the second day. This dish freezes well. Put portions in small zippered freezer bags. Reheat slowly in the microwave. Serves a crowd.

ROXY'S ZUCCHINI PESTO QUICHE

For homemade pesto, see Diane's Basil Pesto, p. 118.

PREPARATION

Preheat the oven to 375°. In a large bowl mix the zucchini, pesto, Parmesan cheese, Monterey Jack cheese, red pepper, eggs, and half and half. Fill the pie crusts with the zucchini mixture, and top with Swiss cheese. Bake for 30 minutes. Serves 6.

INGREDIENTS

3 small zucchini, grated in processor and zucchini liquid squeezed out in a towel

2 tablespoons pesto sauce (fresh or prepared)

½ cup grated Parmesan cheese

½ cup grated Monterey Jack cheese

½ cup finely chopped red bell pepper

3 eggs, beaten

1 cup half and half

2 Marie Callendar's frozen pie crusts

¾ cup grated Swiss cheese

GLAZED CARROTS

INGREDIENTS

1 pound carrots, peeled and grated in processor

1 cup chicken broth

4 tablespoons butter

2 onions, grated in processor

1 tablespoon all-purpose flour

Salt and pepper to taste

Dash nutmeg

⅛ teaspoon sugar

PREPARATION

In a saucepan steam or boil the grated carrots in the chicken broth until very tender, about 10 minutes. In a skillet melt the butter then stir in the onions and sauté for about 5 minutes. Add the flour to the onions and cook for 2 more minutes. Add the carrots and broth, salt, pepper, nutmeg, and sugar. Cook over medium heat until the liquid is thick. Serves 6 to 8.

MARY'S COUNTRY BEAN PÂTÉ

We like to spread a thin layer of pâté on a whole wheat tortilla and cover with thin slices of Muenster cheese. Place in the toaster oven until the cheese is just melted. Remove from the oven, fold the tortilla in half, cool slightly, and slice into triangles. We eat them as a finger food for lunch or snacks.

PREPARATION

In a food processor mince the onion and garlic. Add the beans, breadcrumbs, mustard, lemon juice, oil, ½ teaspoon pepper, nutmeg, parsley, basil, thyme, dill, and tarragon. Process until smooth, stopping once or twice to scrape the mixture down the sides of the work bowl. Adjust the seasonings and add salt and pepper to taste. Cover and refrigerate. Will stay fresh in the refrigerator for about 2 weeks. Use as a spread. Makes about 3 cups.

INGREDIENTS

½ small red onion, diced

2 cloves garlic

1 16-ounce can cannellini beans, drained and rinsed

¾ cup white breadcrumbs

1 teaspoon coarse brown mustard

1 tablespoon lemon juice

1 tablespoon olive oil

½ teaspoon pepper

¼ teaspoon nutmeg

2 tablespoons minced fresh parsley

1 tablespoon minced fresh basil

½ teaspoon each thyme, dill, and tarragon

Salt and pepper to taste

INGREDIENTS

- 1 cup all-purpose flour
- 1 cup plus 2 tablespoons whole milk
- 3 eggs
- 2 tablespoons unsalted butter, browned and cooled
- 1 teaspoon salt
- 2 tablespoons each minced fresh parsley, chives, and tarragon
- Vegetable oil for the crêpe pan (1 teaspoon for each crêpe)

Filling:
- 2 tablespoons olive oil
- ½ onion, minced
- 1 pound mushrooms, chopped

Sauce:
- ⅔ cup soft cream cheese or goat cheese
- ¾ cup vegetable broth, heated
- 2 teaspoons fresh lemon juice
- 1 teaspoon minced garlic
- Salt and white pepper to taste

MUSHROOM CRÊPES WITH GOAT CHEESE SAUCE

PREPARATION

In a blender or food processor combine the flour, milk, eggs, butter, and salt, and process until smooth, turning off the machine and scraping the sides of the container once while mixing. Transfer to a bowl, mix in the herbs, and let stand, covered, at room temperature for 1 hour.

Oil an 8-inch Teflon crêpe pan over medium heat. Add 2 tablespoons of batter and swirl to coat the bottom of the pan. Cook until lightly brown, about 45 seconds. Turn the crêpe over and cook for 30 seconds more. Place the cooked crêpe on a sheet of waxed paper. Repeat, oiling the pan for each crêpe and putting a layer of waxed paper between each crêpe. Can be refrigerated for a few days or frozen for up to a month (wrap well in plastic). Makes about 15 crêpes.

To make the filling, in a skillet heat the oil and sauté the onion until transparent. Add the mushrooms and continue sautéeing until the mushrooms give up their liquid. Set aside.

In a medium bowl whisk together all of the ingredients for the sauce. Warm slightly. Keeps well in the refrigerator.

To assemble the crêpes, on a plate place a portion of warm mushroom filling on a warm crêpe, fold over, and pour warm sauce on top. This recipe is a knockout for special occasions. Crêpes can also be assembled in a 9 x 13-inch glass baking dish for a party and warmed gently in the oven. Guests may serve themselves, pouring warmed goat cheese sauce on top from a gravy boat. Serves 8.

2   medium beets
¼   cup tahini (a paste
    made from toasted
    sesame seeds, found
    in the natural foods
    section of the
    grocery store)
¼   cup fresh lemon juice
1   clove garlic, crushed
½   cup plain yogurt
    Salt to taste

BEETS IN TAHINI AND YOGURT

This Lebanese dish is a colorful and tasty accompaniment to any meal and also serves as a dip for pita bread. The tahini provides a nutty taste without the danger of choking. Does not stick to the roof of the mouth like other nut butters.

PREPARATION

Chop off the tops of the beets. Don't peel. In a saucepan cover the beets with water and cook until tender, about 40 minutes. While running cold water over the beets, rub off the skins with your fingers. Grate in the food processor. In a medium bowl mix the tahini, lemon juice, garlic, yogurt, and salt. Fold in the grated beets. Can be served cold or warm. Serves 6 to 8.

2

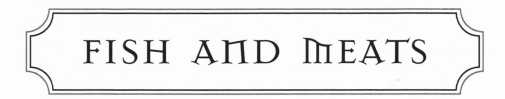

FISH AND MEATS

SALMON PÂTÉ

INGREDIENTS

Casing:

1 tablespoon Dijon mustard

1 tablespoon butter

1 tablespoon lemon juice

Garlic salt, pepper, and dill to taste

1 small piece of fresh salmon (about ½ pound)

½ cup whipped cream cheese

Tabasco sauce to taste

PREPARATION

To make the casing, combine the mustard, butter, lemon juice, garlic salt, pepper, and dill. Melt slightly in the microwave. Place the salmon, skin side down, on a piece of aluminum foil and cover with the mustard casing, reserving some for the dip. Bake in a small toaster oven at 350° until fork tender, about 30 minutes. Remove the skin (it will stick to the foil). In a medium bowl mix the salmon, cream cheese, Tabasco sauce, and the reserved leftover casing mix with a fork until creamy. Serve as a dip with crackers. Makes about 2 cups.

SALMON LOAF WITH CREAMED PEAS

PREPARATION

Preheat the oven to 350°. Generously butter a loaf pan. In a medium mixing bowl beat the egg. Add the breadcrumbs, lemon juice, mustard, cayenne, turmeric, melted butter, sage, and salt. Add the salmon and onions and mix very well. Press into the prepared loaf pan and bake for about 45 minutes. Cool slightly. Remove from the pan and cut into slices. Cook the peas according to package directions, and add to the Basic White Sauce. Place a slice of salmon loaf on each plate, and pour the sauce on top. Serves 4 to 6.

INGREDIENTS

1   egg
¾   cup breadcrumbs
    Juice of ½ lemon
1   tablespoon Dijon mustard
    Dash cayenne pepper
¼   teaspoon turmeric
2   tablespoons melted butter
½   teaspoon sage
    Salt to taste
1   15-ounce can salmon with juice or 1 pound baked fresh salmon
¼   cup minced onions
1   1-pound package frozen peas
1   recipe Basic White Sauce (see p. 110)

INGREDIENTS

Fillets of your favorite flaky white fish, such as halibut, flounder, or tilapia

2 tablespoons white wine per fillet

Dash lemon juice per fillet

Garlic salt and pepper to taste

Fresh herbs, if available, to taste

Pat of butter for each fillet

Sauce:

Liquid from fish pouches

1 tablespoon cornstarch for each cup of liquid

¼ cup white wine

Lemon peel for garnish

QUICK–BAKED WHITE FISH WITH WINE SAUCE

PREPARATION

Place each fillet separately on a piece of aluminum foil, folding up the edges slightly. Pour a little wine and lemon juice over each fillet. Sprinkle garlic salt, pepper, and herbs over each fillet. Place a pat of butter on each fillet before wrapping loosely but securely in a foil pouch. Place in the toaster oven or regular oven at 375° for about 20 minutes, until the fish is flaky but still moist. Remove the fish from the foil. To make the sauce, pour the reserved baking juices into a small saucepan. In a small bowl stir the cornstarch into the wine, add to the reserved juices, and cook on medium heat, whisking constantly, until the sauce is the desired thickness. Serve each fillet on a small bed of cooked spinach, pouring wine sauce on top. Garnish with a few slivers of lemon peel. Goes well with Pesto Mashed Potatoes (see p. 8), because the delicate green color contrasts nicely with the fish.

STEAMED MUSSELS

PREPARATION

Discard mussels that are already opened. Heat a saucepan, then add the wine, garlic, shallots, and mussels. Cover and simmer over medium heat for 5 minutes. Take out the mussels and increase the heat, reducing the liquid by half. Whisk in the cream and butter. Throw in the parsley. Place the mussels in a flat soup bowl, cover with sauce, and sprinkle the top with shaved hard cheese. Can be served with bread dipped in sauce. Serves 4 to 6.

INGREDIENTS

8   ounces white table wine
1   garlic clove, crushed
2   shallots, minced
2   pounds mussels, cleaned
¼   cup whipping cream
1   tablespoon butter
    Chopped parsley
    Hard cheese

INGREDIENTS

- 4 tablespoons butter
- 1 leek, sliced (use all the white and half the green part)
- ¼ cup white wine or vermouth
- 2 tablespoons all-purpose flour
  Salt and pepper to taste
- 1 pound bay scallops
- ½ cup cream

CLAUDIA'S BAY SCALLOPS S IN WHITE WINE

PREPARATION

In a saucepan heat 2 tablespoons butter and sauté the leek for 2 minutes. Add the white wine, cover, and simmer until tender, about 10 minutes. Cool slightly and purée in the processor or blender.

Place the flour, salt, and pepper in a small bag and toss the scallops (pour off and save the liquid first). In a skillet melt the remaining butter and brown the scallops for 4 to 5 minutes, turning to brown on all sides. Add the puréed leeks and wine and reserved juice. Cook for 2 minutes. Stir in the cream. Serve over orzo or fine noodles. Serves 4.

CRAB QUICHE

For those with difficulty swallowing the crust, individual portions of filling may be baked in small ramekins in the same manner as the quiche.

PREPARATION

In a medium bowl cut the butter into the salt and flour using a pastry blender or two sharp knives until the butter pieces are the size of small peas. In a small bowl whisk the egg and ice water together and add to the flour mixture, mixing with a fork. Turn out onto a waxed paper–covered surface and knead with the heel of your hand until the pastry is smooth and holds together in a ball. Roll out and fit into the bottom and sides of a 9-inch pie plate. Patch where needed. No need to be fussy here. Refrigerate.

Preheat the oven to 375°. In a skillet heat the butter and sauté the onions until tender. Line the unbaked pie shell with ¼ cup grated Swiss or Gruyère cheese. Cover with the crab meat. In a large bowl mix the cream, eggs, onions, sherry, and tomato paste. Make a paste with flour and a little of the liquid. Add the paste to the liquid and mix well. Season with salt, pepper, cayenne, and nutmeg, and pour the mixture over the crab meat. Cover with the remaining grated cheese. Bake for about 30 minutes in the lower third of the oven, until the filling has puffed and the top is brown. If refrigerated, let the quiche come to room temperature, then bake for 15 minutes or so in a 375° oven. Let stand for 20 minutes before serving. Serves 6 to 8.

INGRE

Crust:

1   stick unsalted butter (cold)

⅛   teaspoon salt

1½ cups unbleached flour

1   egg

2   tablespoons ice water

Filling:

2   tablespoons melted butter

2   tablespoons minced shallots or green onions

½   cup grated Swiss or Gruyère cheese

1½ cups crab meat

1   cup light cream

4   eggs, beaten

2   tablespoons dry sherry or dry vermouth

1   tablespoon tomato paste

1   tablespoon flour

⅛   teaspoon salt
    Pepper
    Pinch cayenne pepper

¼   teaspoon nutmeg

INGREDIENTS

GRILLED FILET MIGNON AND PORTOBELLO MUSHROOMS

- 1 portobello mushroom per filet
  Olive oil
- 1 filet mignon per person
- 1 white onion, chopped
- 2 cloves fresh garlic, chopped
  A-1 or Worcestershire sauce

PREPARATION

Remove the stems carefully from the mushrooms and remove the brown part. Brush with olive oil (mushrooms absorb liquid easily, so don't soak). Grill the steaks as usual, grilling the mushrooms as you would the steak, about 8 minutes on each side. Meanwhile, in a skillet heat some olive oil and sauté the onion and garlic. Add a little A-1 or Worcestershire sauce for more flavor. Put one steak (for the person with swallowing difficulties) in the processor with some of the juices from the steak, and pulse for just a brief moment. Pile the steak on the mushroom and cover with sautéed vegetables. Prepare the guests' steaks by slicing mushrooms and placing under or around steak.

MACHACA CON HUEVOS (SHREDDED BEEF WITH EGGS)

PREPARATION

In a skillet heat 1 tablespoon oil and brown the beef strips. Set aside. In a large saucepan combine the water, wine, chiles, cinnamon stick, orange peel, green onions, and ginger. Bring to a boil, add the beef, and simmer, covered, until the beef is tender, about 1 hour 30 minutes (or 6 hours in a crock pot). Remove the cinnamon stick and orange peel strips. Cool, then shred the meat (or pulse in the processor), saving the cooking liquid. Use about one-fourth of the meat for Machaca con Huevos and freeze the remainder.

In a large skillet heat 2 tablespoons vegetable oil and sauté the onion, bell pepper, jalapeño pepper, and tomato until very tender. Add the beef and beaten eggs and move gently until the eggs are set. Stir in the Mexican cheese. To prepare, wrap the meat mixture in a tortilla and cover with salsa verde. Serve with your favorite potatoes. This is good for brunch too. Serves a crowd.

INGREDIENTS

1   tablespoon oil
1½ pounds tri-tip pot roast, cut into strips
1   cup water
½   cup red wine
¼   teaspoon crushed red chiles
1   cinnamon stick
    Strips of orange peel
2   green onions, sliced
    Fresh ginger
2   tablespoons vegetable oil
½   small onion, diced
½   green bell pepper, diced
    Small piece of jalapeño pepper, minced
1   fresh tomato, chopped
4   eggs, beaten
½   cup Mexican cheese
    Corn tortillas
    Salsa verde (found in Mexican food section of grocery)

LITTLE HAM LOAVES

- 1 1½-pound pork steak, ground in the processor
- 1 1-pound ham steak, ground in the processor
- 1 cup breadcrumbs (made from stale whole wheat bread pulsed until fine in the processor)
- 1 cup milk
- 2 eggs, beaten
  Pepper

Sauce:
- 1½ cups brown sugar
- ½ cup vinegar
- ½ cup water
- 1 teaspoon dry mustard

PREPARATION

Preheat the oven to 375°. In a large bowl mix the pork, ham, breadcrumbs, milk, eggs, and pepper. Roll into small loaves (oval-shaped, about 2 x 4 inches) and place in a 9 x 13-inch baking dish. Bake for 15 minutes.

Meanwhile, make the sauce. In a large saucepan combine all of the ingredients for the sauce, and boil for 5 minutes. Reduce the oven temperature to 350° and bake the ham loaves for 30 minutes more, basting with sauce every 5 minutes. Serves 6 to 8.

PULLED PORK BBQ

PREPARATION

Place the roast in a slow cooker. In a medium bowl mix the other ingredients and pour over the roast. Cook for 6 to 8 hours. Remove the roast and cool. Pull into shreds with a fork, or pulse 3 times in the processor (1 second on, 1 second off). *Note:* Put no more than 2 cups of roast in the processor at a time. Use the liquid from the slow cooker in processing. Toss the pork with your favorite barbecue sauce. Serve with coleslaw or Braised Red Cabbage (see p. 20) and refried beans. Serves a crowd.

INGREDIENTS

1 2½-pound shoulder or butt roast (bone-in) tied or netted
¼ cup bourbon
1 tablespoon molasses
¾ cup cider vinegar
1 cup water
1 teaspoon salt
2 teaspoons red pepper
2 teaspoons black pepper

VANESSA'S GREEN CHILE CHICKEN ENCHILADAS

INGREDIENTS

- 1 whole roasting or frying chicken
- 1 bunch green onions, minced
- 8 ounces sour cream
- 1 4-ounce can diced green chiles
- 2 8-ounce bags grated Mexican cheese (Kraft), or ½ pound each grated Asadero and queso blanco (see description of queso blanco under Breakfast Burrito, p. 61)
- ½ cup peanut oil
- 1 dozen corn tortillas
- 1 28-ounce can green chile enchilada sauce

PREPARATION

Preheat the oven to 350°. In a large pot cover the chicken with water and simmer for about 2 hours. Cool the meat and pull from the bone. Chop coarsely in the food processor in two batches. Pulse at rate of 1 second on, 1 second off until the chicken is coarsely chopped (about 4 pulses). In a large bowl mix the chicken, onions, sour cream, green chiles, and three-fourths of the cheese, and set aside. In a medium fry pan heat the peanut oil on medium heat and fry the tortillas, one at a time, on each side until tender (about 15 seconds on each side), placing on paper towels to absorb the oil. Pour a little enchilada sauce into the bottom of a 9 x 13-inch baking dish, then assemble the enchiladas. Place a handful of the chicken mixture on each tortilla, roll, and place snugly in the pan. Top with the remaining enchilada sauce and cheese. Bake for 30 minutes to warm through and melt the cheese. Top each serving with Guacamole (see p. 116) if desired. Leftovers freeze well. Serves a crowd.

CHICKEN TAMALE PIE

PREPARATION

Preheat the oven to 350°. Grease a 2-quart casserole. In a mixing bowl prepare the muffin mix according to package directions and stir in the Cheddar cheese. Set aside. In a saucepan combine the soup, chili powder, garlic, chiles, onions, corn, and turkey until blended and heat through. Spoon the muffin mixture into the prepared casserole. Spoon the hot mixture over the muffin mixture to within ½ inch of the edge. Bake for 25 minutes, until the corn bread is golden. Garnish with additional cheese, green onions, and sliced cherry tomatoes if desired. Serves 6.

INGREDIENTS

1 12-ounce package corn muffin mix

½ cup shredded Cheddar cheese

1 can cream of chicken soup

1 teaspoon chili powder

1 clove garlic, minced

1 4-ounce can chopped green chiles

½ cup chopped green onions

1 cup whole kernel corn

1½ cups cooked shredded turkey, or ground in processor

Green onions and cherry tomatoes for garnish

INGREDIENTS

1   chicken, whole or pieces
1   onion, quartered
4   cloves garlic
6   sprigs each of fresh thyme, oregano, and parsley
1   recipe Mole Sauce (see p. 111)

CHICKEN WITH MOLE SAUCE

PREPARATION

In a large pot cover the chicken with water and add the onion, garlic, sprigs of thyme, oregano, and parsley. Bring to a boil, reduce the heat, and simmer until tender, about 45 minutes.

Add a little chicken broth to the Mole Sauce and pour over the stewed chicken (shred to desired consistency). Cook for about 20 minutes, uncovered. The sauce should be thick. Serve with tortillas and refried beans or Orzo (see p. 3) mixed with Cilantro Pesto (see p. 118). Serves a crowd.

KENTUCKY–STYLE STEWED CHICKEN AND DUMPLINGS

PREPARATION

In a large pot cover the chicken with water. Add the bay leaf, clove, carrots, celery, onion, garlic, parsley, and salt and pepper to taste. Cover and simmer slowly until the chicken is tender, about 1 hour. Remove the chicken and carrots from the water. Discard the bay leaf.

Into a medium bowl sift together the flour, baking powder, and salt. Cut in the butter with two knives or a pastry cutter until the mixture has the consistency of meal (the butter is almost invisible). Add the milk to make a soft dough (don't mix too much). Turn onto a floured surface and roll as thin as possible (paper thin). Cut into 1- to 2-inch squares. Drop the squares into the boiling chicken liquid, cover, reduce the heat, and simmer for 20 minutes without opening the lid. Scoop the dumplings from the liquid with a slotted spoon and serve in a bowl with some cooking liquid to keep the dumplings from sticking together. Serve with the chicken and carrots. Accompany with blended coleslaw and cranberry sauce. Freeze the remaining cooking liquid for future use. Serves 8 to 10.

INGREDIENTS

1 chicken, cut into pieces (use all parts)
1 bay leaf
1 whole clove
3 to 4 carrots, peeled and cut into large pieces
1 large celery stalk, sliced (use tops)
1 onion, chopped
3 cloves garlic
¼ cup chopped Italian parsley
   Salt and pepper to taste

Dumplings:
2 cups all-purpose flour
1½ teaspoons baking powder
1 teaspoon salt
1 tablespoon butter
⅔ cup milk

CHICKEN OR TURKEY À LA KING

INGREDIENTS

1 recipe Basic White Sauce (see p. 110)

2 tablespoons dry sherry

¼ teaspoon dill weed

2 tablespoons butter

¼ onion, grated

½ green and/or red pepper, grated

¼ pound mushrooms, finely chopped

½ pound tender chicken or turkey, cooked and shredded or ground, depending on desired consistency

1 cup petite peas, if tolerated

PREPARATION

To the Basic White Sauce, add dry sherry and dill. In a saucepan melt the butter and sauté the onion, green pepper, and mushrooms until tender. Add to the sauce. Add the shredded meat and peas. Cook until hot. Serve over biscuits or mashed potaotes. Serves 6.

CHICKEN LIVER PÂTÉ

When liverwurst won't do.

PREPARATION

In a saucepan melt 1 tablespoon butter. Add the onion and sauté for 1 minute, then cover and cook for about 10 minutes until quite soft. Cut the livers into quarters. In a skillet heat the oil and add the livers. Sprinkle with salt and pepper, and cook on high heat for a few minutes, turning to cook on all sides. Remove from the skillet. In the same skillet melt the remaining tablespoon of butter and add the livers and onions. Sprinkle with the sage and cook, stirring, for about 3 minutes. Sprinkle with cognac and ignite it. Cool slightly and purée in the processor, using the metal blade. Shape by pressing into a ramekin, then turning out onto a plate. Serve at room temperature or cold with crackers and a nice merlot. Serves 6.

INGREDIENTS

2   tablespoons butter
⅓   cup minced onion
½   pound chicken livers
3   tablespoons oil
     Salt and pepper to taste
½   teaspoon ground sage
1   tablespoon cognac

INGREDIENTS

2 tablespoons olive oil

Lamb steaks, shoulder, or leg (about 2½ pounds)

1 onion, sliced

3 fresh garlic cloves, minced

1 28-ounce can tomatoes, cut into pieces

Strips of orange peel and juice of 1 orange

½ cup red or white wine

2 tablespoons curry powder

1 large eggplant, peeled and cut into small cubes

Petite peas, almonds, yogurt, and chutney for garnish

BRAISED LAMB AND EGGPLANT PROVENÇALE

PREPARATION

Preheat the oven to 325°. In a large ovenproof pot heat the olive oil and brown the lamb pieces. Remove the meat and sauté the onion and garlic until tender. Add the tomatoes, orange juice and peel, wine, curry powder, and eggplant. Place the meat on top of the vegetable mixture, cover, and bake for 2 hours. After 1 hour, remove from the oven to stir the contents, covering the meat with the vegetables, and return to the oven. Before serving, remove the orange peel. Serve over fine egg noodles. Top with peas, sliced almonds (or ground in the processor), a dollop of yogurt, and chutney. For the person with swallowing difficulties, the lamb may be pulsed briefly in the processor and topped with the eggplant mixture. Serves 8.

SHEPHERD'S PIE

PREPARATION

Preheat the oven to 425°. In a medium skillet melt the butter and sauté the onion and mushrooms. Remove from the skillet and brown the lamb. Add the water, gravy mix, Worcestershire sauce, salt, pepper, and onion mixture. Put into a 9 x 13 x 2-inch baking dish. In a mixing bowl beat the potatoes and egg together until smooth. Spread over the lamb mixture. Bake for 20 minutes. Serves 6.

INGREDIENTS

- ¼ cup butter
- 1 onion, chopped
- 4 ounces mushrooms, sliced
- 1 pound lamb, ground
- 1 cup water
- 1 packet brown gravy mix
- 2 teaspoons Worcestershire sauce
- ½ teaspoon salt
- ¼ teaspoon pepper
- 2 cups mashed potatoes
- 1 egg

INGREDIENTS

MOUSSAKA

¼ cup olive oil

1 pound lean lamb, ground

1 large onion, finely chopped

1 clove garlic, minced

¼ teaspoon ground cinnamon

1 teaspoon salt

⅛ teaspoon each nutmeg and white pepper

¼ teaspoon dried oregano

¼ cup chopped parsley

2 tablespoons tomato paste

½ cup dry red wine

1½ pounds eggplant, peeled and thinly sliced

½ cup freshly grated Parmesan cheese

Cream Sauce:

2 tablespoons butter

2 tablespoons flour

½ teaspoon salt

  Dash nutmeg and white pepper

2 cups milk

2 eggs

1 egg yolk (save egg white to add to scrambled eggs)

PREPARATION

In a large frying pan heat 1 tablespoon olive oil and brown the lamb. Mix in the onion and cook until tender. Mix in the garlic, cinnamon, salt, nutmeg, white pepper, oregano, parsley, tomato paste, and wine. Bring to a boil, reduce the heat, cover, and simmer for 15 minutes. Uncover and continue simmering until the sauce is thick, about 5 minutes. Arrange the eggplant slices on a cookie sheet in a single layer. Brush with some of the remaining oil, and broil about 4 inches from the heat until lightly browned, about 5 minutes. Turn, brush the other side, and broil the same way.

Preheat the oven to 350°. To assemble, place half of the eggplant slices in a single layer in an ungreased 2-quart casserole. Top with the meat mixture. Sprinkle with 2 tablespoons Parmesan cheese. Cover with the remaining eggplant and 2 tablespoons cheese.

To make the sauce, melt the butter in a medium saucepan. Stir in the flour, salt, nutmeg, and white pepper. Remove from the heat and gradually stir in the milk. Return to the heat and cook, stirring, until thick. In a small bowl beat the eggs and yolk. Mix in a little of the heated sauce. Over low heat, whisk the egg mixture gradually into the sauce. Pour the sauce over the casserole. Sprinkle with the remaining Parmesan cheese. Bake until the top is lightly browned, about 45 minutes to 1 hour. Serves 8.

BREAKFAST DISHES

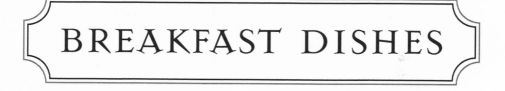

There are more breakfast ideas in Chapter 7, Desserts and Fruits. Also included here are a few favorite easy-to-eat breakfast bread recipes. Egg dishes are also included here, although eggs make a great meal any time.

CREAM OF WHEAT

PREPARATION

Hot cereal made from scratch tastes so much better than instant package mix and doesn't take much longer to prepare. Prepare with milk instead of water for added nutrition. Experiment with cooking times to get the right texture for easy chewing and swallowing. Avoid oatmeal, which doesn't form a bolus, or mass, in the mouth. Try combinations of these additions: brown sugar, maple syrup, butter, soaked raisins or prunes, half and half, or cream. Mix in fresh processed strawberries for great color and added texture.

POACHED EGG WITH HOLLANDAISE SAUCE ON GRITS

PREPARATION

There are many ways to poach eggs. This is our favorite. Put salted water in a heavy pan and heat to boiling. Slide each egg into the pan from a saucer. Keep the heat low and don't let the water boil while the eggs cook. To "cover the eye," when the egg is about cooked ladle some of the hot water on top of the yolk. Remove the eggs one at a time with a slotted spoon. Prepare Easy Blender Hollandaise Sauce (p. 113). Prepare grits according to package directions, making a fairly thick texture. Place the grits in a flat soup bowl, forming a well in the center. Place the cooked egg in the well and pour the warm Hollandaise sauce on top.

Variation: Make a bed for the poached egg in chopped cooked spinach. Cover with Hollandaise sauce.

INGREDIENTS

CHEESE SOUFFLÉ

- 2 cups milk
- 3 tablespoons butter
- 3 tablespoons minced shallots
- 4 tablespoons all-purpose flour
  Salt and pepper to taste
- ⅛ teaspoon nutmeg
  Pinch of cayenne pepper
- 2 teaspoons cornstarch
- 1 tablespoon water
- 6 large eggs, separated
- ¼ cup finely grated Parmesan cheese
- ¼ pound Swiss or Gruyère cheese, grated

PREPARATION

Preheat the oven to 375°. Butter a 5-cup soufflé dish. In a saucepan bring the milk to just short of boiling. In another saucepan melt the butter and sauté the shallots until tender. Add the flour, stirring with a whisk. While stirring, add the hot milk, salt, pepper, nutmeg, and cayenne, and cook for about 5 minutes. In a small bowl blend the cornstarch and water and add to the pan. Remove from the heat and add the egg yolks, whisking rapidly. Add the grated Parmesan cheese. Move the mixture to a large bowl. Beat the egg whites until stiff, and fold into the mixture with a spatula. Fold in the Swiss or Gruyère cheese. Pour into the prepared soufflé dish. Bake for about 20 minutes, until puffed and golden. Serves 6.

DEVILED EGGS

PREPARATION

In a pan cover the eggs with water, bring gently to a boil, cover, and turn off the heat. Let the pan sit on the burner for 10 to 15 minutes until the eggs are hard-boiled. Drain and run cold water over the eggs. Shake the eggs in the pan until the shells crack and loosen, then peel. Slice the eggs in half lengthwise. Remove the yolks to a small bowl and mix with the mayonnaise, dry mustard, vinegar, Worcestershire, Tabasco, garlic salt, white pepper, and onion. Fill the egg whites with the yolk mixture. Sprinkle the eggs with paprika if desired. Use any leftover yolk mixture as an egg dressing (add a little melted butter to thin) for vegetables, such as asparagus. Serves a crowd.

6 eggs
2 tablespoons mayonnaise
½ teaspoon dry mustard
1 teaspoon vinegar
   Dash Worcestershire sauce
   Dash Tabasco sauce (optional)
   Garlic salt and white pepper to taste
2 tablespoons finely minced onion, or 1 teaspoon sweet pickle relish
   Paprika for garnish (if desired)

INGREDIENTS

½ cup Grape Nuts
2 cups milk
½ cup sugar
1 egg, beaten
½ teaspoon vanilla

VANESSA'S GRAPE NUTS GLIDER

PREPARATION

Preheat the oven to 300°. In a baking dish soak the Grape Nuts in the milk for 30 minutes. Add the sugar, egg, and vanilla. Bake, uncovered, for 1 hour. Serve warm or cold, topped with half and half or milk if desired. Leftovers taste great reheated. Serves 6 to 8.

GRAHAM CRACKER RENNET CUSTARD

PREPARATION

Dissolve the rennet tablet in the water. In a saucepan heat the milk and honey slowly, stirring until warm (a drop on the inside of your wrist feels slightly warm). Overheating will destroy the rennet. Place 1 graham cracker in the bottom of each of 4 dessert cups. Mix the dissolved rennet into the warm milk and pour into the dessert cups. Let set for 10 minutes without moving, then refrigerate. Serves 4.

INGREDIENTS

1   rennet tablet

2   tablespoons water

2   cups milk

¼   cup flavorful honey (lavender is good)

4   graham crackers (2½-inch squares)

INGREDIENTS

POTATO FRITTATA

This is an open-faced omelet. You can add just about any vegetable to a frittata—whatever's around. Shred and sauté them along with the potatoes and onions.

¼ cup olive oil

1 medium potato, peeled and shredded with the shredder blade of the processor

¼ onion, shredded

¼ red or green pepper, shredded

4 eggs, beaten (Use the reserved egg whites for meringue or to add to scrambled eggs for more protein.)

1 teaspoon fresh minced rosemary or other spice

Grated cheese

PREPARATION

In a large heavy skillet heat the olive oil and fry the potato, onion, and pepper until tender, about 10 minutes. Pour in the eggs and rosemary and cook over low heat until the bottom is golden, about 5 minutes. To cook the top, place a plate on top of the pan and carefully turn the omelet over onto the plate, then slide back into the pan. Sprinkle your favorite grated cheese on top, and cook until set, just a minute or so. The omelet should be moist, not dry. Leftovers make great take-along snacks. Put a piece in a zippered bag. Tastes good at room temperature, and can be reheated in a microwave and topped with salsa. Serves 6.

BISCUITS AND GRAVY

PREPARATION

In a small saucepan mix the flour with the drippings and cook for a few minutes, until slightly brown. Add the milk gradually, stirring with a whisk until smooth. Add the thyme and pour over freshly baked biscuits. (Make biscuits from scratch or use the ready-to-bake variety.) Serves 4 to 6.

INGREDIENTS

2 tablespoons all-purpose flour

2 tablespoons drippings from bacon or breakfast sausage

1 cup milk

1 tablespoon fresh thyme and/or sage, minced

FRENCH TOAST

INGREDIENTS

1 egg for each slice of bread, beaten

A little milk

Dash of nutmeg or cinnamon and/or a drop or so of vanilla

Slices of your favorite bread with the crusts cut off

Butter

Pure maple syrup or puréed fruit, such as strawberries or mangoes

PREPARATION

In a shallow dish combine the eggs, milk, and spices. Soak the bread until as much of the mixture as possible is absorbed. On a skillet or griddle melt butter and fry the bread until golden brown on each side. Serve with warm maple syrup or puréed fruit.

BREAKFAST BURRITO

Experiment with a variety of Mexican cheeses for a great-tasting burrito. Queso fresco is usually made from a combination of cow's and goat's milk and tastes like a mild feta cheese. It crumbles easily. Queso blanco is a creamy white cheese made from skimmed cow's milk. It becomes soft and creamy when heated but it doesn't melt. This is an ideal stuffing for burritos.

PREPARATION

If using hash browns, cook according to package directions and mix into the scrambled eggs. If using refried beans, spread a small amount in a horizontal strip in the center of each warm tortilla, then place the eggs on top. Sprinkle the cheese and salsa on top. Fold the lower end of the tortilla over the strip of filling, fold the sides over, then fold the top over. To serve or keep warm, wrap in foil. *Note:* Tofu may be added to or substituted for scrambled eggs. Press the desired amount through a ricer and scramble with the eggs. Serve with sour cream and guacamole if desired.

INGREDIENTS

Frozen hash brown potatoes (optional)

Eggs, scrambled in butter with salt and pepper to taste (1 egg for each tortilla)

Canned refried beans (optional), heated

Soft wheat tortilla, warmed (wrap in foil and heat in a toaster oven at 250° for a few minutes)

Mexican cheese, such as queso fresco or queso blanco, shredded

Salsa (in Mexican food or refrigerated section of grocery)

Sour cream and guacamole (if desired)

PANCAKES

PREPARATION

Make your favorite pancake batter and add thinly sliced bananas to the top of the pancake before turning. Adding shredded apple, crushed pineapple, or whole blueberries to the batter also provides texture and variety to a one-dimensional food. Add fresh grated lemon rind to the batter for great flavor. Cottage cheese added to the batter provides an interesting texture and flavor, as does replacing milk with buttermilk or yogurt. Adding a pinch of cinnamon or nutmeg is great too. Serve with warm pure maple syrup. Keep pancakes warm in the oven while cooking. Freeze unused pancakes by placing a sheet of waxed paper between each one, then wrapping tightly in plastic or a zippered plastic bag. Rewarm on low heat in the toaster oven or in the microwave.

MOM'S POOR MAN'S FRUITCAKE

PREPARATION

Preheat the oven to 325°. Oil and flour 2 1-pound loaf pans. In a large mixing bowl mix the raisins, cold water, oil, sugar, spices, and salt. Sift the flour and baking soda together and add to the raisin mixture. Beat well. Pour into the prepared loaf pans and bake for 1 hour.

Let cool on a rack for 20 minutes before removing from the pans. Cool completely before slicing. To serve, spread a layer of cream cheese on each slice.

INGREDIENTS

1 pound raisins, stewed 15 minutes in 2 cups water and cooled

1 cup cold water

½ cup oil

2 cups sugar

1 teaspoon cinnamon

1 teaspoon cloves

1 teaspoon nutmeg

1 teaspoon salt

4 cups all-purpose flour

1 tablespoon baking soda

Cream cheese (optional)

EASY APPLESAUCE BREAKFAST BREAD

INGREDIENTS

- 1 stick butter
- ½ cup granulated sugar
- ½ cup brown sugar
- 2 eggs
- 1 cup applesauce
- 1½ teaspoons baking soda
- 2 cups all-purpose flour
- ½ teaspoon salt
- 2 teaspoons ground cardamom
- ½ teaspoon ground nutmeg
- ½ teaspoon ground ginger
- ¼ teaspoon ground cloves

PREPARATION

Preheat the oven to 375°. Grease and flour a 1-pound loaf pan. In a large bowl cream the butter and sugars. Add the eggs. Stir in the applesauce. In a medium bowl combine the dry ingredients and add to the moist ingredients. Put into the prepared loaf pan and bake for about 50 minutes. Cool for a few minutes, then remove from the pan and set on a rack until cool.

MUSHROOM AND/OR HAM SOUFFLÉ

PREPARATION

Preheat the oven to 350°. In a skillet melt the butter and sauté the mushrooms (or ham) and onion until tender. In a small bowl beat the egg yolks and blend into the Basic White Sauce. Add the mushroom-ham mixture. In a medium bowl beat the egg whites until stiff and fold into the mixture. Pour into an ungreased casserole and set in a pan of hot water. Bake for about 40 minutes or until a knife inserted into the center comes out clean. Serves 6.

INGREDIENTS

2 tablespoons butter

½ pound mushrooms, chopped, or ¼ pound ham, ground in the processor to the desired consistency

¼ onion, minced

3 eggs, separated

1 recipe Basic White Sauce (see p. 110)

INGREDIENTS

ALICE'S SIX-WEEK MUFFINS

3 cups bran cereal (raisin bran, rice bran, oat bran flakes, etc.)
1 cup sugar
2½ cups flour
1 tablespoon baking soda
1 teaspoon salt
1 teaspoon cinnamon
2 cups mashed ripe banana or 1 8-ounce can crushed pineapple
2 eggs
½ cup vegetable oil
2+ cups buttermilk

PREPARATION

In a large bowl mix the dry ingredients together. Add the remaining ingredients and mix well. Cover and refrigerate for at least 6 hours.

Preheat the oven to 400° (for large muffins) or 350° (for small muffins). Grease (or use paper baking cups) and almost fill the muffin tins.

Bake large muffins for 18 to 20 minutes; bake small muffins for 12 to 15 minutes. Store the batter in the refrigerator for up to six weeks. Makes 24 large or 60 small muffins.

BANANA BRAN BREAD

PREPARATION

Preheat the oven to 350°. Grease a 1-pound loaf pan. In a mixing bowl beat together the butter and sugar until creamy. Beat in the egg, vanilla, and bran flakes. In a blender process the bananas, grated orange rind, and orange juice concentrate until smooth. Sift the dry ingredients together and add to the blender alternately with the moist ingredients until mixed thoroughly. Bake in the prepared loaf pan for 1 hour. Place on a rack for about 20 minutes, then remove from the loaf pan. Allow to cool completely before slicing. Slices taste great spread with cream cheese.

INGREDIENTS

¼ cup butter, softened

½ cup sugar

1 egg

1 teaspoon vanilla

1 cup Raisin Bran flakes

1½ cups very ripe bananas (about 3 small bananas)

1 tablespoon grated orange rind (optional)

2 tablespoons frozen orange juice concentrate

1½ cups flour

2 teaspoons baking powder

½ teaspoon salt

½ teaspoon baking soda

4

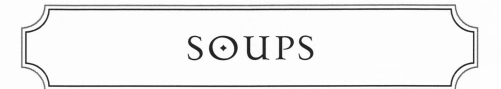

SOUPS

YIN YANG SOUP (DARK AND LIGHT)

INGREDIENTS

2 tablespoons olive oil
1 onion, chopped
2 cloves garlic, chopped
2 15-ounce cans black beans, not drained
1 15-ounce can tomatoes or one fresh tomato, chopped
1 stalk celery, chopped
1 carrot, chopped
½ sweet pepper (green, red, yellow), chopped
1 4-ounce can diced mild green chiles or 1 tablespoon chopped jalapeño chile
1 tablespoon cumin or chili powder
1 bay leaf
1 teaspoon dried oregano or sweet basil, or 1 tablespoon chopped fresh oregano or basil
3 tablespoons chopped fresh cilantro
   Juice of 1 lime
   Salt and pepper to taste
   Sour cream or crème fraîche

YIN: SOUTHWESTERN BLACK BEAN SOUP

PREPARATION

In a large pot heat the olive oil and sauté the onion and garlic until tender. Add the beans, tomatoes, celery, carrot, sweet pepper, chiles, cumin, bay leaf, and oregano, and simmer until the vegetables are tender, about 45 minutes. Remove from the heat and cool slightly. Purée in the blender in two or three batches. Add fresh cilantro while blending. Pour back into the pot and squeeze in the lime juice. Add salt and pepper to taste. Should be hot and spicy. Serve with a dollop of sour cream or crème fraiche. Serves 8.

This soup reflects in taste and appearance the Chinese Yin and Yang principle of the interaction of opposites. The spicy black bean soup and sweet corn soup complement each other when tasted together in each spoonful. Of course each soup can be eaten alone, but the presentation of the two soups together is a real hit with guests.

YANG: SWEET CORN SOUP

PREPARATION

In a large pot melt the butter and sauté the onion and potato for 1 minute. Add 1 cup broth, cover, and simmer for 5 minutes. Add the corn and remaining broth, simmering until tender, about 15 minutes (a little longer for fresh corn). Remove from the heat and cool slightly. Add the spices and purée in the blender in two batches. Pass through a food mill to remove the hulls, which might cause choking. Add a little half and half if the soup is too thick or you desire a richer soup. Serves 8.

To serve, pour both soups slowly at once into a flat soup bowl (like a pasta bowl). Carefully add a dollop of sour cream or crème fraîche to the bean soup and a dollop of bean soup to the corn soup to complete the yin yang symbol. Freeze unused portions of soups separately in small zippered bags.

INGREDIENTS

1 tablespoon butter

½ onion or 1 to 2 shallots, chopped

1 potato, peeled and grated

5 cups chicken broth, chicken stock, or water

6 ears yellow corn, kernels sliced off cob, or 4 15-ounce cans yellow kernel corn, drained

Fresh or dried spices (of your choice)

Half and half (optional)

BRIE SOUP

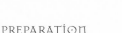

½ cup butter

6 leeks, sliced (use all the white and a little of the green part)

4 cups unsalted chicken stock

½ cup all-purpose flour

4 cups half and half

1½ pounds cold ripe Brie with rind

White pepper

PREPARATION

In a skillet melt ¼ cup butter. Add the leeks and sauté for 4 minutes. Add the stock, bring to a boil, reduce the heat and simmer, covered, for 25 minutes. Cool slightly and purée in the blender in two batches. Meanwhile, in a stock pot (not aluminum) combine ¼ cup butter and the flour. Cook and stir for 2 minutes. Add the half and half, one cup at a time. Add the Brie in chunks, and cook on medium heat, stirring until the cheese is melted (the rind will still be in pieces). Pass the Brie mixture through a food mill or strainer and discard the rind. Mix the Brie with the puréed leeks. Add white pepper to taste. This soup is best if refrigerated overnight. Reheat slowly before serving. Goes well with Poached Pears (see p. 134) and a crisp white wine. Serves 8.

ASPIC (JELLIED SOUPS)

Canned bouillon and canned consommé can easily be turned into aspic. For soup, use 1 envelope of gelatin for 3 cups of liquid. For molded aspics, use 1 cup of gelatin for 2 cups of liquid. Sprinkle the gelatin into ¼ cup of cold liquid and let it soften for 3 minutes. Blend it into the rest of the liquid and stir over medium heat for several minutes until the gelatin is completely dissolved. See the recipe below for one example of jellied soup.

JELLIED BEEF CONSOMMÉ

PREPARATION

To remove the skin from the tomato, plunge it into boiling water for 1 minute. The skin should peel away easily. Purée the tomato in the blender. In a large pot bring the broth to a boil and add the tomato and wine. Remove from the heat. Dissolve the gelatin in the water, and add to the pot along with a splash of lemon juice. Chill until set. Break the consommé apart and serve in small bowls. It is also good hot, but the consistency will be thinner and not as easy to control in swallowing. Serves 6 to 8.

INGREDIENTS

1 ripe tomato

3 cups beef bouillon or broth

¼ cup Madeira wine (optional)

1 envelope unflavored gelatin

¼ cup cold water

Splash of lemon juice

MOLDED TOMATO ASPIC

PREPARATION

- ½ cup shredded cabbage
- ½ cup finely diced celery
- 2 tablespoons diced onion
- 1 15-ounce can stewed tomatoes
- 2 1-ounce packages unflavored gelatin
- ¼ cup cold water
- ¼ cup sugar
- 1 teaspoon dry mustard
- 1 teaspoon salt
- ¼ cup vinegar
- 2 tablespoons diced stuffed olives
  Mayonnaise for garnish

In a large pot cook the cabbage, celery, and onion in the tomatoes until the vegetables are tender. Dissolve the gelatin in the cold water, and add to the hot tomatoes, stirring until totally dissolved. Cool slightly and purée in the blender. Mix in the sugar, mustard, salt, and vinegar. Pour into a 5-cup mold and add the olives. Chill until firm. Unmold by immersing in cold water for about 30 seconds. Turn over onto a serving plate. Accompany with a small dollop of mayonnaise on each serving. Serves 6 to 8.

CLAM JUICE CONSOMMÉ

PREPARATION

In a saucepan heat the clam juice and chicken broth. Remove from the heat and beat the egg yolks into the hot broth, stirring vigorously with a whisk. Stir in the wine, cream, and pepper. Serve hot or cold. Serves 6 to 8.

INGREDIENTS

2   cups bottled clam juice

1   cup chicken broth

3   egg yolks, beaten (Use the reserved egg whites for meringue or to add to scrambled eggs for more protein.)

    Splash of white wine

¼   cup cream

    White pepper

INGREDIENTS

1 potato, peeled and diced into small cubes
1 stalk celery, diced
1 quart milk or half and half
1 bay leaf
2 tablespoons all-purpose flour
2 tablespoons water
1 teaspoon salt
¼ teaspoon pepper
1 pint oysters (use liquor) or ⅔ cup crab meat or lobster, pulsed a few times in processor if required
¼ cup butter

OYSTER, CRAB, OR LOBSTER BISQUE

PREPARATION

In a saucepan place the potato, celery, milk, and bay leaf, and heat to scalding. Remove the bay leaf. Make paste of the flour, water, salt, and pepper. Combine with the oysters in a saucepan and simmer over low heat for about 10 minutes. Add to the hot milk mixture. Add the butter. Cover and let stand for 15 minutes before serving. Drop a piece of butter into serving dishes and pour the hot soup over. Serve with oyster crackers. If serving at a party, keep the soup warm in a crock pot. Serves 6.

LESLIE'S ZUCCHINI BISQUE

PREPARATION

In a saucepan heat the olive oil and sauté the onion, garlic, and bell pepper on low heat until tender. Add the zucchini and chicken broth and cook slowly until the vegetables are very tender. Season with fresh herbs, white pepper, VegSal, and lemon juice. Cool slightly and purée in the blender or food processor. To serve, dollop with sour cream, buttermilk, or yogurt. Serves 8.

INGREDIENTS

¼ cup olive oil

1 medium onion, sliced

1 large clove garlic, minced

1 green bell pepper, chopped

4 medium zucchini, chopped

1 14-ounce can chicken broth

¼ cup fresh herbs (parsley, oregano, etc.)

White pepper and VegSal (seasoned salt) to taste

Juice of ½ lemon

Sour cream, buttermilk, or yogurt for garnish

LEE'S CUCUMBER SOUP

1 cucumber, peeled (remove seeds if they cause swallowing difficulty) and chopped

½ cup chopped onion

½ cup plain yogurt or sour cream

Juice of ½ lemon

¼ teaspoon cumin

½ teaspoon dill weed

Salt and pepper to taste

PREPARATION

In the processor or blender purée all of the ingredients until smooth. Chill. Serves 3 to 4.

VARIATION: BEET SOUP

PREPARATION

Use 2 medium beets in place of the cucumber. Remove the beet tops. Before combining the ingredients in the processor, cover the unpeeled beets with water in a small pan and cook for about 40 minutes, until the skins peel off easily with the thumb (cool first!). Also tastes fine heated. Serves 3 to 4.

EASY BEET SOUP

PREPARATION

Blend the pickled beets (you'll find the best at a farmers' market) and yogurt or buttermilk in the blender. Drain and discard the pickle juice for a thicker soup, which is easier to swallow. If tart foods cause a problem, rinse the beets in water before processing. Serve cold or hot.

INGREDIENTS

1   15-ounce jar prepared pickled beets

½   cup yogurt or buttermilk

INGREDIENTS

- 1 1-pound bag dried peas
- 2 tablespoons olive oil
- 1 onion, diced
- 1 carrot, diced
- 1 stalk celery, diced
- ½ pound (approximately) ham hocks or salt pork
- 1 14-ounce can chopped tomatoes
- 2 tablespoons chili powder
- 2 cloves garlic, minced
- ¼ cup chopped parsley
- 1 teaspoon minced fresh marjoram
- 1 teaspoon minced fresh rosemary
- 1 teaspoon minced fresh thyme
- 2 bay leaves

SPLIT PEA SOUP WITH HAM

PREPARATION

In a large bowl cover the peas with water. In a large pot heat the olive oil and sauté the onion, carrot, and celery. Drain the peas and add to the pot with 6 cups of water. Add the salt pork or ham hocks. Simmer until tender, about 2 hours. Add the cut tomatoes, chili powder, garlic, parsley, marjoram, rosemary, thyme, and bay leaves. Remove the bones and fat. Cool slightly. Remove the bay leaves. Purée the soup, including the ham (2 cups at a time) in the processor. Add more water while processing if the soup becomes too thick. Serves a crowd.

ASPARAGUS LEMON SOUP

PREPARATION

In a saucepan cook the asparagus, leek, and potato in the broth until the vegetables are tender, about 20 minutes. Cool slightly and purée (pass through a food mill or strainer to remove any fibers). Return to the heat and add the cream, salt, pepper, lemon juice, and nutmeg, and heat until warm (don't boil). Garnish with grated lemon peel. This soup is great with shrimp and egg salad and a crisp chardonnay. Serves 4 to 6.

INGREDIENTS

1   pound fresh asparagus, chopped (break off and discard tough ends)

1   leek, chopped (use the white and some of the green)

1   small potato, peeled and cooked

3   cups broth

½   cup whipping cream

Salt and white pepper to taste

Juice of 1 small lemon and grated peel

Dash nutmeg

ALICE'S CHILLED AVOCADO SOUP

- 4 large avocados, peeled, pitted, and cut into chunks
  Juice of 1 lemon
- 2 cups plain yogurt (regular or low-fat)
- ¼ teaspoon Tabasco sauce
- 2 cups milk
- 3 scallions, trimmed and chopped
- 2 cloves garlic, peeled and chopped
- 1 red bell pepper, sliced crosswise, for garnish
- 6 tablespoons sour cream for garnish
  Fresh or dried cilantro for garnish

PREPARATION

In the processor combine the avocado chunks and lemon juice. Blend until smooth. Add the yogurt, Tabasco sauce, milk, scallions, and garlic, and blend until smooth. Refrigerate at least 1 hour before serving. Serve in chilled bowls garnished with red pepper slices, sour cream, and cilantro. Consume the day of preparation. Does not keep well. Serves 6.

POTATO LEEK SOUP (VICHYSSOISE)

Called vichyssoise if served cold.

PREPARATION

In a 5-quart pot cook the potatoes, leeks, broth, wine, salt, pepper, and bay leaves until the vegetables are very tender, about 25 minutes. Cool slightly and remove the bay leaves. Purée in the processor using the metal blade, 2 cups at a time. Return to the pot and add the half and half. Heat carefully without boiling. If serving cold, sprinkle finely cut fresh chives on top before serving to enhance the flavor. (Well-cooked diced carrots, turnips, cauliflower, broccoli, or zucchini may be added if soft foods can be tolerated, or if other diners prefer more texture.) Serves 6 to 8.

INGREDIENTS

2 pounds potatoes, peeled and quartered (use boiling, not baking potatoes)

2 leeks, cut into 1-inch pieces (use all of white and half of green part)

3½ cups broth

½ cup dry white wine

1 teaspoon salt

¼ teaspoon pepper

2 bay leaves

1½ cups half and half

EGG DROP SOUP

INGREDIENTS

4 cups chicken broth
2 teaspoons dry sherry
2 teaspoons soy sauce
1 clove garlic, minced
1 1-inch piece ginger, minced
2 cups diced spinach leaves (or a bunch of watercress if you have it)
2 eggs
Salt to taste

PREPARATION

In a 2-quart pan heat the chicken broth, sherry, and soy sauce to boiling. Add the garlic and ginger. Add the spinach and simmer, uncovered, for 2 minutes. In a small bowl beat the eggs lightly. Remove the pan from the heat and pour the eggs slowly into the soup, whisking constantly, until they form threads. Season with salt. Serves 8.

BANGKOK BUTTERNUT SQUASH SOUP

PREPARATION

Cut the squash in half and scoop out the seeds. Place facedown in a glass baking dish and cover with plastic wrap, lifting one corner to let out steam. Microwave on high for about 10 minutes, or until very tender. Let cool, then scoop out the flesh, discarding the rind. In a large pot melt the butter over medium heat and sauté the onion, garlic, and ginger until tender. Stir in the Thai curry paste and cook for 1 minute. Add the squash, chicken stock, coconut milk, salt, and pepper. Bring to a boil, reduce the heat, and simmer for 20 minutes. Cool slightly, then puree in two batches in the blender or processor. To thin, add more broth. To thicken, add mashed potato flakes or potato starch. Stir in the lime. Serve hot in a flat bowl with a dollop of crème fraiche. Serves 8.

INGREDIENTS

1 small butternut squash

1 tablespoon butter

1 small onion, chopped

2 cloves garlic, minced

1 tablespoon minced fresh ginger

½ teaspoon Thai red curry paste (be careful, this is hot)

2 cups chicken stock

1 cup coconut milk, light or regular

1 teaspoon salt

1 teaspoon pepper

Juice of 1 lime

Crème fraîche for garnish

(*Note:* Williams-Sonoma carries a jar of Butternut Squash purée that can be used in place of fresh.)

INGREDIENTS

PEANUT SOUP

2 teaspoons peanut oil or vegetable oil

2 tablespoons finely chopped onion

1 clove garlic, minced

1 teaspoon fresh ginger, minced

1 package Thai peanut sauce mix (international food section of grocery store)

1 14-ounce can coconut milk (regular or light)

¼ cup creamy peanut butter

2 cups chicken broth

6 tablespoons (approximately) instant mashed potatoes

PREPARATION

In a saucepan heat the oil and sauté the onion, garlic, and ginger for a few minutes. Add the Thai peanut sauce mix, coconut milk, peanut butter, and chicken broth. Add the instant mashed potatoes (a little at a time until the desired consistency is achieved), cooking and stirring for a few minutes until hot and thick. Serves 4.

MARY'S NO HASSLE REFRIED BEAN SOUP

PREPARATION

In a saucepan mix the ingredients and heat. Makes a great thick base for soup. Depending on consistency level desired, you can add raw zucchini or summer squash, processed into small pieces and cooked to desired tenderness; sour cream or buttermilk; or shredded chicken. Serves 6 to 8.

INGREDIENTS

1   14-ounce can refried beans (regular or black bean)

1   14-ounce can stewed tomatoes (low-salt)

1   14-ounce can vegetable broth (low-salt)

INGREDIENTS

LEBANESE LENTIL SOUP

Look for colorful lentils, which provide a soup with more eye appeal than ordinary brown lentils.

1 cup red (or pale orange) lentils, washed and drained

6 cups water

1 onion, chopped

1 carrot, chopped

½ cup chopped celery tops

½ cup chopped cilantro leaves

1 vegetable bouillon cube

2 teaspoons cumin

Salt and pepper to taste

2 teaspoons butter

Juice of ½ lemon

Plain yogurt for garnish

PREPARATION

Place the lentils in a soup pot with the water. Bring to a boil, and add the onion, carrot, celery tops, cilantro, and bouillon cube. Lower the heat and simmer until the lentils fall apart, about 45 minutes. Cool slightly and pass the soup through a food mill or strainer. Return to the pot and reheat, adding the cumin, salt, pepper, butter, and lemon juice. Serve with a generous dollop of yogurt. Serves a crowd.

CREAM OF MUSHROOM SOUP

PREPARATION

In a saucepan over medium heat melt the butter and sauté the mushrooms, garlic, and onions until the mushrooms give up their liquid, about 7 minutes. Whisk in the flour and cook for 1 minute. Then stir in the hot chicken broth, bay leaf, and herbs, whisking constantly and cooking until thick, about 1 minute. Remove bay leaf and discard. Stir in the half and half, salt, and pepper. Pulse in the processor if necessary for puréed consistency. Add a little white wine if desired to make a thinner texture. Goes well with liver pâté or liverwurst. Serves 4.

INGREDIENTS

- 2 tablespoons butter
- ½ pound mushrooms, chopped
- 1 clove garlic, minced
- ¼ cup chopped onions
- 2 tablespoons all-purpose flour
- 1½ cups hot chicken broth
- 1 bay leaf
- ⅛ cup your favorite fresh herbs
- 1 cup half and half
  Salt and pepper to taste

ALICE'S FRENCH ONION SOUP

- ¼ cup butter
- 1 clove garlic, crushed
- 6 cups sliced onions (about 4 large onions)
  Pepper to taste (white pepper recommended)
- 1 quart vegetable stock (or water)
- 2 tablespoons miso dissolved in 2 cups hot water
  Tamari Soy Sauce to taste
- ½ cup white wine
- 6 or more thin slices of day-old French bread, toasted
  Grated Swiss cheese

PREPARATION

Preheat the oven to 400°. In a saucepan melt the butter and sauté the garlic and onions over medium heat until very well done, 45 minutes or so, stirring often. It's good if they stick to the pan a little and brown. Add the pepper and wet ingredients. Ladle into ovenproof soup bowls. Place a piece or two of toasted French bread on top to cover the soup. Cover with grated Swiss cheese. Place in the oven and bake until the cheese is brown and bubbly. Cool slightly before serving. Makes 6 large bowls.

TRACY'S CHICKEN ENCHILADA SOUP

PREPARATION

In a large pot heat the oil and sauté the onion and garlic until translucent. Add the chicken broth. In a medium bowl combine the masa harina with 2 cups water and whisk until blended. Add the mixture to the pot. Add remaining water (if desired), chicken, enchilada sauce, Velveeta, and spices to the pot and bring to a boil. Reduce heat and simmer about 30 minutes until thick. Remove from the heat and add the lime juice. Soup may be puréed for easier chewing and swallowing. Just before serving, place a dollop of cold guacamole on top of each bowl. For diners without swallowing problems, corn kernels may be added to the bowl for texture (delicious use of leftover corn). Freezes well. Serves 10 to 12.

INGREDIENTS

- 1 tablespoon vegetable oil
- 1 cup diced onion
- 1 clove garlic, pressed
- 1 quart chicken broth
- 1 cup masa harina (find in the flour section or Hispanic foods section of the grocery store)
- 2 to 3 cups water, depending on desired thickness
- 1 pound (approximately 2 cups) shredded cooked chicken breasts
- 1 cup red enchilada sauce (use mild if affected person reacts to hot foods)
- 1 pound Mexican-style Velveeta cheese
- 1 teaspoon chili powder
- ½ teaspoon cumin
  Juice of 1 lime
  Guacamole (optional)
  Whole kernels of cooked fresh white corn cut from the cob (optional)

CREAM OF BROCCOLI SOUP

INGREDIENTS

1 tablespoon vegetable oil
1 small onion, chopped
4 cups fresh broccoli, chopped (remove small leaves as they are bitter)
2 cups chicken broth
1 cup ricotta cheese
1 cup milk
  Juice of ½ lemon
  Salt and pepper to taste
¼ cup grated Parmesan cheese

PREPARATION

In a saucepan heat the oil and sauté the onion for a few minutes. Add the broccoli and broth, bring to a boil, reduce the heat, cover, and simmer for about 20 minutes until the broccoli is very tender. Remove from the heat and cool slightly. In a blender combine the ricotta cheese and milk until smooth. Add to the soup. Stir in the lemon juice, salt, and pepper. Purée in two batches in the blender. Return to the saucepan and heat slowly, but do not boil. Stir in the Parmesan cheese before serving. Serves 6 to 8.

SPIΠACH AΠD POTATO SOUP

PREPARATIOΠ

In a large saucepan melt the butter and sauté the scallions and spinach for 1 minute. Mix in the flour, add the broth, potatoes, and spices, and simmer until the potatoes are soft, about 10 minutes. Cool slightly. Purée in the blender in two batches. Add the lemon juice. Add a dollop of crème fraîche on top of each serving. Serves 4.

IΠGREDIEΠTS

1 tablespoon butter

1 bunch scallions, sliced (use green part too)

1 10-ounce bag spinach leaves

1 tablespoon all-purpose flour

1 quart vegetable broth

4 potatoes, peeled and cubed

Fresh spices, such as parsley, dill, or cilantro to taste

Juice of ½ lemon

Crème fraîche for garnish

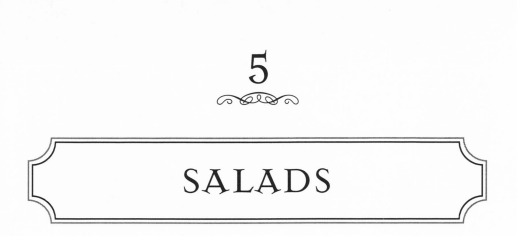

5

SALADS

BLENDED SALAD

Blended salad has all the freshness and flavor of salad without the hassle of major chewing. You can fix salads at home to take to outings, but don't give samples, or you won't have any left for yourself!

PREPARATION

Put your favorite vegetables in the food processor. Sample combo: half a tomato, half a peeled cucumber, half an onion, a sturdy lettuce like romaine, a green pepper (red pepper makes the salad brown), a fresh squeeze of lemon, your favorite salad dressing (Honey Dijon vinaigrette is good). Pulse in the processor, 1 second on and 1 second off, about 3 or 4 times until you achieve the desired consistency. Overblending creates mush. Serve with crackers as a dip. Eating crackers with the salad helps to form a bolus for easier movement in the mouth. Make only enough to eat now because this salad tastes best when fresh.

COLESLAW

PREPARATION

Process the cabbage, onion, and carrot using the shredding blade. Mix in the remaining ingredients (you can vary the amounts to your own taste). Goes well with chicken and dumplings. Serves about 8.

INGREDIENTS

½ head cabbage

¼ onion

1 carrot

½ cup mayonnaise (see recipe for homemade, p. 112)

¼ cup sugar

¼ cup buttermilk

¼ cup white vinegar

Salt and pepper to taste

CRAB LOUISE

A takeoff on Crab Louis.

INGREDIENTS

1 10-ounce bag spinach greens, steamed
2 cups shredded crab meat
2 hard-cooked eggs, finely chopped
2 tablespoons minced or grated onion
1 fresh tomato, peeled (place in boiling water for 1 minute, then skin will come off easily)
1 avocado, peeled

Dressing:

1 cup mayonnaise (see recipe for home-made, p. 112)
½ cup chili sauce
½ cup unsweetened whipped cream
   Juice of ½ lemon
   Tapénade (olive spread; see the recipe on page 100 or use prepared variety) for garnish

PREPARATION

Arrange the spinach on 4 small plates and mound ½ cup crab meat in the center of each. In a small bowl mix the chopped egg and onion and sprinkle one-fourth of the mixture over the crab meat. Arrange thin slices of tomato and avocado around the outside of the plates, alternating vegetables. In a small bowl mix the mayonnaise, chili sauce, whipped cream, and lemon juice, and pour over the salad. Place a dollop of tapénade on top of each arrangement. Serves 4.

EGG SALAD

PREPARATION

In a large bowl combine all of the ingredients. Mix well. Tastes great served with a dollop of tapénade (olive paste) for added zing. Tapénade can be purchased ready-made in gourmet food shops, or follow the easy recipe on the next page. Serves 6 to 8.

4   hard-cooked eggs, shelled and finely chopped

2   tablespoons finely diced onion, or 1 teaspoon onion powder

2   tablespoons finely diced celery, or 1 teaspoon celery seed, or 1 teaspoon celery salt

2   tablespoons pickle relish

½   cup mayonnaise (see recipe for homemade, p. 112)

Salt and white pepper to taste

Dash of dill weed

VARIATION: SHRIMP SALAD

PREPARATION

Add minced or processed shelled, cooked, and cooled shrimp to Egg Salad. Serves 8.

TAPÉNADE

INGREDIENTS

1   cup pitted olives (I like Greek kalamata olives, but anything works, especially mixed varieties)

¼   cup capers, rinsed (optional)

2   garlic cloves

2   teaspoons minced fresh thyme

    Fresh ground pepper to taste

    Fresh lemon juice to taste

2   tablespoons extra virgin olive oil

PREPARATION

In the food processor combine the olives, capers, garlic, thyme, pepper, and lemon juice, and make a relatively smooth paste, adding the olive oil through the feeder tube while the machine is running. Tastes great as a topping for Crab Louise or Egg Salad (see pp. 98–99). Keeps well in the refrigerator for about 3 weeks.

HAM SALAD

PREPARATION

In a medium bowl mix all of the ingredients. Serve on crackers or small cocktail bread (find in the deli section of the grocery store). Serves 6 to 8.

INGREDIENTS

1   ½-pound ham, grated in processor (pulse 1 second on, 1 second off until desired consistency)

2   hard-boiled eggs, grated in processor

½   teaspoon dry mustard

¼   teaspoon pepper

⅛   cup celery, grated in processor

⅛   cup onion, grated in processor

½   cup mayonnaise

2   tablespoons sweet relish (optional)

INGREDIENTS

MACARONI SALAD

Drippings from 3 slices bacon

1 tablespoon minced onion

⅛ cup each minced green pepper and celery

1 tablespoon vinegar

Salt and pepper to taste

¼ teaspoon prepared mustard

¼ cup mayonnaise

½ cup very small elbow macaroni, cooked until tender

PREPARATION

In a skillet heat the bacon drippings and fry the onion, green pepper, and celery until tender. Add the vinegar, salt, pepper, mustard, and mayonnaise, and mix well. Add the macaroni and adjust the seasonings. Tiny squares of soft cheese, such as Danish Havarti, may be added for texture. Serves 6.

TUNA SALAD WITH CONCHIGLIETTE AND PEAS

PREPARATION

In a medium bowl mix the tuna, egg, onion, celery, relish, salt, pepper, dill, and mayonnaise. Carefully fold in the macaroni and peas. Serve chilled. For those without eating problems, the tuna mixture can be served in a hollowed-out fresh tomato. For the affected person, chop the scooped-out tomato portion into small pieces and arrange on top of a scoop of salad. Avocado slices arranged decoratively on top looks festive. Makes a great luncheon dish. Serves 4.

Vegan mayo —

INGREDIENTS

1 small can albacore tuna packed in water, drained

1 egg, hard-boiled and finely chopped

1 tablespoon finely diced onion, or onion powder if small pieces cause choking

1 tablespoon finely diced celery, or celery seed if small pieces cause choking

1 tablespoon pickle relish

Salt and pepper to taste

Dash of dill weed

½ cup mayonnaise (see quick homemade variety on p. 112)

½ cup cooked conchigliette (small macaroni shells), cooled

½ cup cooked petite peas

1 small fresh tomato for each serving

1 ripe avocado

INGREDIENTS

2 tablespoons olive oil
1 cup minced onions, or shredded in processor
½ teaspoon curry powder
¼ teaspoon cinnamon
¼ teaspoon cumin
Pinch of turmeric
¾ cup chicken broth
3 cups carrots, shredded in processor
3 cups cooked whole wheat couscous
½ cup currants, softened by boiling gently in ¼ cup water until plump
½ cup pine nuts, toasted (300° on a baking sheet in the toaster oven for about 5 minutes; watch carefully or they will burn in an instant) and ground in the processor
Zest of 1 lemon
Salt and pepper to taste
¼ cup minced fresh mint

LOIS'S CURRIED CARROT COUSCOUS WITH CURRANTS

Because couscous is made of very small pieces and forms a bolus (or mass) well, this grain makes a dish that is easy to chew and not likely to cause choking.

PREPARATION

In a large saucepan heat the olive oil and cook the onions for 3 minutes. Stir in the curry, cinnamon, cumin, and turmeric. Cook another minute. Add the chicken broth and carrots. Cover and cook for about 10 minutes, until the carrots are very tender. Place the couscous in a large bowl and toss. Add the onion and carrot mixture and the currants (with cooking liquid), pine nuts, and lemon zest. Toss again. Add salt and pepper. Cool. Toss with the mint, cover, and refrigerate. Makes a great dish to take to a picnic. Serves 8 to 10.

FRUIT SALAD

PREPARATION

Process fresh fruits, such as high antioxidant strawberries or blueberries (don't process these two
together unless you like purple food!), with a little
confectioners' sugar, which dissolves quickly.
Makes a great topping for ice cream, pancakes,
tapioca pudding, etc. Optional: Add Grand
Marnier, cognac, Framboise, or other favorite
liqueurs. Keeps well in the refrigerator for about 1
week.

INGREDIENTS

MOLDED AMBROSIA SALAD

1   3-ounce package apricot-flavored gelatin

1   cup boiling water

½   cup white wine, chilled

½   cup cold water

5   ounces frozen sliced strawberries, thawed (use liquid)

½   cup crushed pineapple (use liquid)

1   banana, peeled, cut in half lengthwise, and sliced

½   cup sour cream

1   tablespoon brown sugar

PREPARATION

In a heatproof bowl stir the gelatin into the boiling water for 2 minutes until dissolved. Add the wine and cold water and chill until partially set. Stir in the strawberries, pineapple, and banana. Pour into a greased mold or small custard cups. Cover and chill for at least 3 hours. In a small bowl combine the sour cream and brown sugar, and serve with the salad. Serves 4.

CRANBERRY MOLD

PREPARATION

In a heatproof bowl dissolve the gelatin in the hot water. Add the syrup from the pineapple can and sugar. Chill until partially set. Add the cranberries, apple, and pineapple. Pour into individual molds or ramekins and refrigerate until firm. Unmold if desired. Serves 4.

INGREDIENTS

1   3-ounce package lemon-flavored gelatin

1   cup hot water

1   8-ounce can crushed pineapple in syrup (use syrup)

1   cup frozen cranberries, ground (or 1 cup jellied cranberry sauce if smoother consistency is desired)

1   cup ground apple

1   cup sugar

6

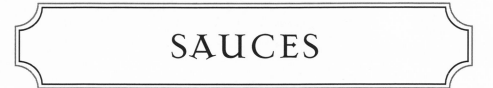

SAUCES

INGREDIENTS

- 3 tablespoons butter
- 3 tablespoons all-purpose flour
- 2 cups milk
  Salt and pepper to taste

BASIC WHITE SAUCE (BECHAMEL)

Adds flavor, moisture, and texture to meats, vegetables, salads, and desserts.

PREPARATION

In a saucepan melt the butter and add the flour, stirring constantly over medium heat for 2 minutes. Remove from the heat. Pour the milk slowly into the flour mixture, stirring with a whisk. Return to the heat, whisking until thickened. Add salt and pepper to taste. Great on cauliflower, broccoli, or cabbage, or as a base for scalloped potatoes.

VARIATION: CHEESE SAUCE

PREPARATION

For Cheese Sauce, stir in ½ cup sharp Cheddar cheese to the finished Basic White Sauce.

MOLE SAUCE

You can buy mole (MOH-lay) sauce in the Mexican foods section of the grocery store, but homemade is the best. Tastes great on chicken.

PREPARATION

Remove the stems from the chiles and cut in half lengthwise to remove the seeds. Toast briefly in a hot skillet, then cover with hot water in a small bowl. Peel the tomatoes and discard the skin. Pulse in the processor a few times. In a skillet toast the sesame seeds until just brown. Add to the processor with the tomatoes, along with the oregano, clove, and allspice. Process until smooth. Add the oil to the skillet and fry the onion pieces until translucent, then add the garlic cloves and cinnamon stick and fry for a few more minutes. Transfer to the processor, leaving the oil in the skillet. Fry the plantain or banana for a few minutes and transfer to the processor along with the chiles and water. Process until smooth. Strain the sauce through a food mill and return to the skillet. Add the chocolate and season with salt.

INGREDIENTS

12 chiles guajillos (wa-HEE-yos), cleaned

3 ripe tomatoes or tomatillos, peeled

¼ cup sesame seeds

1 tablespoon dried oregano

1 whole clove

½ teaspoon allspice

¼ cup oil

1 small onion, quartered

8 cloves garlic

Large piece of cinnamon stick

1 plantain or firm banana, peeled and chopped

1 ounce Mexican chocolate (Ibarra or Abuelito brand)

Salt to taste

1 large egg

2 tablespoons cider vinegar

½ teaspoon dry mustard

½ teaspoon salt

2 to 3 fresh garlic cloves, minced

1 cup vegetable oil

LOIS'S HOMEMADE MAYONNAISE

You're probably going to be eating a lot of this and there's nothing like homemade, especially with a little fresh garlic added. Try egg salad or coleslaw made with fresh mayonnaise and a little dill or as an accompaniment to cold salmon for lunch.

PREPARATION

In a blender combine the egg, vinegar, mustard, salt, garlic, and ¼ cup oil. Turn on the motor and add the rest of the oil in a slow, steady stream. It will thicken as the oil is poured in. Makes 1 cup. Keeps for 1 week in the refrigerator.

EASY BLENDER HOLLANDAISE SAUCE

You'll never buy prepared again.

PREPARATION

In the blender combine the egg yolks, salt, and cream. Cover and blend for 30 seconds. Pour half of the melted butter into the pour cap in a steady stream with the blender on high. Add the lemon juice, then the remainder of the butter, with the blender running. Stop the blender, taste, and add the Tabasco. To keep warm, place the sauce in a bowl of warm water, being careful not to heat too much or the eggs will scramble. Keep the leftovers in the refrigerator for many uses that call for flavored butter. Reheat carefully, or just spoon cold on hot food and allow to melt. Great on asparagus, artichokes, green beans, sautéed spinach, and poached eggs. Makes about 1 cup.

INGREDIENTS

3 egg yolks (reserve whites for scrambled eggs)

½ teaspoon salt

1 tablespoon cream

⅔ cup unsalted butter, melted

1 tablespoon lemon juice

Dash Tabasco sauce

CRÈME FRAÎCHE

1 tablespoon cultured buttermilk

2 cups heavy cream

Crème fraîche is the French version of sour cream (not as sour) and will keep in the refrigerator for about 10 days. It tastes wonderful dolloped on fruits and other desserts, and as a garnish on hot or cold soups.

PREPARATION

In a jar with a lid combine the buttermilk and cream. Cover, shake well, and let stand at room temperature overnight. Refrigerate. Makes a thick cream.

ORANGE–PINEAPPLE SAUCE

Great on fish like orange roughy.

PREPARATION

Peel the orange and slice about half of the peel into julienne strips. In a saucepan heat the olive oil and sauté the garlic, ginger, and orange peel for 1 minute. Add the chicken broth, sugar, juice from the orange, and crushed pineapple (and lemon juice if you like sweet and sour). In a small bowl blend the cornstarch and dry sherry. Add to the sauce, stirring and cooking until the sauce thickens and bubbles slightly. Can be refrigerated for a quick sauce for frozen fish. Makes 2 batches, about ¾ cup in each batch.

INGREDIENTS

1 orange

1 tablespoon olive oil

1 teaspoon diced fresh garlic

1 teaspoon peeled and diced fresh ginger

1 cup chicken broth

2 tablespoons sugar

½ cup crushed pineapple

2 tablespoons lemon juice (optional for tartness)

1 tablespoon cornstarch

1 tablespoon dry sherry

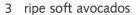

GUACAMOLE

3   ripe soft avocados
½   cup of your favorite
    salsa
⅓   cup sour cream or
    silken tofu (puréed)
    Juice of 1 lime
    Garlic salt to taste

PREPARATION

In a bowl mash the avocados with a fork. Add the salsa, sour cream, lime, and garlic salt, and mix well. Use the food processor for a smoother consistency. A lighter version can be made by substituting fat-free plain yogurt for sour cream. Makes about 2 cups.

MOM'S STEWED TOMATOES

Great over fish or very fine noodles. You can buy stewed tomatoes in a can, but they're not half as good as the way Mom made them.

PREPARATION

Remove the skins from the tomatoes by placing in boiling water for about 1 minute. The skins should peel off easily. In a saucepan cook the tomatoes (crushed) with onion, celery, basil, sugar, salt, and pepper, until the vegetables are very tender, about 25 minutes. Cool slightly and pass through a food mill or processor. In a small bowl mix the cornstarch with a small amount of water and add to the tomatoes, stirring and cooking until slightly thick. Serves 3.

INGREDIENTS

2 large fresh tomatoes

¼ cup finely chopped onion

¼ cup finely chopped celery

Fresh basil leaves

2 tablespoons sugar

Salt and pepper to taste

1 tablespoon cornstarch

INGREDIENTS

INGREDIENTS

- 2 cups tightly packed, washed, and drained basil
- ½ cup or more freshly grated Parmesan cheese
- ½ cup extra virgin olive oil
- 2 large cloves garlic or more to taste
- ¼ to ½ cup toasted pine nuts

DIANE'S BASIL PESTO

Keep a jar of commercially prepared basil pesto sauce in the cupboard for when you don't have fresh basil leaves. This versatile and flavorful sauce can be used as a topping for soups or potatoes, as a sandwich spread, or as a covering for salmon.

PREPARATION

In the processor combine all of the ingredients using the metal cutting blade. Pulse 1 second on and 1 second off a few times until coarsely ground, then scrape the sides of the work bowl. Continue processing until the mixture is a fine consistency. Great with pasta and in Roxy's Zucchini Pesto Quiche (p. 25). Makes about 2 cups.

VARIATION: CILANTRO PESTO

PREPARATION

Follow the recipe for Basil Pesto, but instead of basil use 2 cups cilantro leaves with the thick stems removed. Add the juice of one lemon to add flavor and maintain the bright green color. Cilantro pesto is great mixed into warm orzo or grains, such as bulgar wheat.

7

DESSERTS AND FRUITS

Moist cakes (especially with a dip of ice cream or sauce on top) make for easy eating.
Included in this section are basic recipes for some of our personal favorites. Don't forget
homemade ice creams and sherbets, especially when summer fruits are plentiful. Also, there's
nothing as comforting as cookies dipped in milk.

BASIC VANILLA CUSTARD

INGREDIENTS

2 cups half and half
¼ cup sugar
2 eggs
½ teaspoon vanilla
Grated nutmeg and cinnamon for garnish

PREPARATION

Preheat the oven to 375°. In a small saucepan heat the half and half and sugar over low heat without boiling, until the sugar is dissolved. In a 1-quart pan beat the eggs and gradually whisk in the hot half and half. Stir in the vanilla. Pour the custard into 4 to 6 custard cups. Set the cups in a baking pan. Sprinkle nutmeg and cinnamon on top of each cup. Add warm water to the baking pan to come at least one inch up the sides of the custard cups. Bake until the custard is set, about 35 minutes. Chill. Serves 4 to 6.

BANANAS FOSTER

PREPARATION

In a small skillet melt the butter. Add the sugar and cinnamon. Cook over medium heat until bubbly. Add the banana slices and heat for 3 to 4 minutes, basting constantly with syrup. Pour half of the rum into the skillet. (Remove the rum bottle from the area before igniting.) Ignite the remaining rum in a large spoon by warming the underside of the spoon with a long-handled butane lighter. Pour over the bananas, basting until the flames die down. Serve immediately over ice cream. Serves 2.

INGREDIENTS

2   teaspoons butter
¼   cup brown sugar
    Dash cinnamon (optional)
1   banana, peeled, halved, and sliced lengthwise
¼   cup rum
    Vanilla ice cream

MOUSSE AU CHOCOLAT

INGREDIENTS

- 3 eggs, separated
- 12 teaspoons sugar
- 2 squares unsweetened or semisweet chocolate
- 1 teaspoon hot strong coffee (liquid, not powdered)

PREPARATION

In a medium bowl beat the egg whites until frothy, then while beating gradually add 6 teaspoons sugar until the whites are stiff. In a large bowl beat the egg yolks with 6 teaspoons sugar until thick and light yellow. In a small microwave-safe bowl melt the chocolate in the coffee for a few seconds (watch carefully; you don't want it to bubble) and add to the egg yolks, beating thoroughly. Fold the egg whites into the yolks. Put in individual ramekins and chill for about 8 hours. Serves 6.

FABULOUS FLAN

PREPARATION

Preheat the oven to 300°. In a small saucepan combine 1 cup sugar and ¼ cup water and cook over low heat, whisking frequently, until the sugar melts and becomes golden brown, about 15 minutes. Pour into the bottom of 6 small ovenproof custard cups. In a medium bowl beat the eggs and yolks with the salt and ½ cup sugar until pale yellow. In a saucepan heat the half and half until hot but not boiling. Add to the eggs in a slow stream, whisking constantly. Pour into the custard cups. Place the cups in a baking pan and pour hot water into the pan up to one inch from the top of the cups. Bake until set, about 30 minutes. Cool, then refrigerate for at least 3 hours. To unmold, dip the custard cups into boiling water for about 15 seconds, then turn upside down onto a plate. Serves 6.

INGREDIENTS

Caramel:
1 cup sugar
¼ cup water

Custard:
2 eggs plus 2 yolks
   Dash salt
½ cup sugar
2 cups half and half

CUSTARD KUGEL

- ¼ pound fine noodles
- 1 apple, peeled and sliced or shredded (depending on desired consistency)
- 4 eggs
- 1 stick unsalted butter
- ¼ pound cream cheese
- 8 ounces sour cream
- ½ cup sugar
- 1 teaspoon vanilla
- ⅛ teaspoon nutmeg

PREPARATION

Preheat the oven to 350°. Generously grease a baking dish. Cook and drain the noodles. Line the prepared baking dish with the noodles. Layer the shredded apple on top. In a large bowl blend the eggs, butter, cream cheese, sour cream, sugar, vanilla, and nutmeg. Pour over the noodles. Bake for 1 hour, until brown. Serves 6.

CHOCOLATE CAKE PUDDING

A delicious variation on bread pudding.

PREPARATION

Preheat the oven to 350°. In a large heavy saucepan combine the milk, cream, and sugar over medium high heat until the sugar dissolves and the mixture comes to a boil. Remove from the heat, add the chocolate, and stir until smooth. In a large bowl blend the eggs and vanilla. Gradually whisk in the chocolate mixture. Add the cake cubes and let stand for about 30 minutes, stirring occasionally, until the cake absorbs the mixture. Transfer the mixture to a 9 x 13-inch glass baking dish. Cover with foil and bake for about 45 minutes, until the pudding is set in the center. Serve the pudding warm with warm Bourbon Sauce. Serves a crowd.

INGREDIENTS

2 cups whole milk

2 cups heavy whipping cream

½ cup white sugar

6 ounces Mexican chocolate (find in Mexican food section of grocery store)

8 eggs

1 teaspoon vanilla extract, or Mexican orange liqueur or other orange liqueur

1 pound stale pound cake or any dry cake, cut into 1-inch cubes

BOURBON SAUCE

PREPARATION

In a saucepan heat the sugar, butter, and cream until the sugar is dissolved. Cook over medium heat until smooth and hot, then stir in the bourbon. Serve warm over ice cream, peaches, or bread pudding. Make 2 batches if using as a sauce for Chocolate Cake Pudding.

INGREDIENTS

1 cup light brown sugar, packed

½ cup unsalted butter

½ cup cream

2 teaspoons good bourbon

1 cup graham cracker crumbs (works well in processor)

¼ cup brown sugar

3 teaspoons butter, melted

32 ounces soft cream cheese (8 ounces mascarpone, Italian cream cheese, can replace one cup regular cream cheese for a more delicate taste)

2 teaspoons vanilla

4 eggs

2 1-ounce squares unsweetened chocolate, melted

1¾ cups sugar

MARBLE CHEESECAKE

Some restaurants are known for their cheesecake, but here is a good one that competes well.

PREPARATION

Preheat the oven to 325°. In a bowl mix the graham cracker crumbs, brown sugar, and butter. Press the mixture into a 9-inch square baking pan (or a springform pan if you have one). Place the cream cheese and vanilla in the work bowl of the processor. Using the plastic mixing blade, beat until fluffy, about 2 minutes. Scrape the bowl. While the processor is running, add the eggs one at a time through the feed tube, beating for about 15 seconds after each addition. To melt the chocolate, place in a microwave-safe container and heat in the microwave for about 30 seconds on high (watch carefully; you don't want it to bubble). Remove and stir until melted, then cool for a few minutes. Stir in the sugar. Pour one-third of the cream cheese mixture into a small bowl and whisk in the melted chocolate. Pour the plain and chocolate batter alternately onto the graham cracker mix. Swirl lightly with a knife. Bake for 1 hour and 30 minutes. Cool on a rack for 30 minutes. Refrigerate for at least 2 hours. To serve, cut into squares. If using a springform pan, remove the form and slice. Serves a crowd.

BLACK RUSSIAN BUNDT CAKE

Pudding cakes are very moist and easy to make. We like this one. It's so moist and flavorful, with an "adult" taste.

PREPARATION

Preheat the oven to 350°. Grease and flour a bundt pan. In a bowl combine the sugar, chocolate pudding mix, cake mix, salad oil, eggs, water, vodka, and ¼ cup Kahlua, and beat for 4 minutes. Pour the batter into the prepared pan. Bake for 45 to 50 minutes. Let cool on a rack for 20 minutes before removing from the pan.

To make the frosting, in a small bowl combine the confectioners' sugar with ¼ cup Kahlua. Mix well. When the cake is completely cool drizzle the frosting on top. Serves 10 to 12.

INGREDIENTS

½ cup sugar

1 3-ounce package instant chocolate pudding mix

1 package yellow cake mix

1 cup mild salad oil

4 eggs

¾ cup water

¼ cup vodka

¼ cup Kahlua

Frosting:

½ cup confectioners' sugar

¼ cup Kahlua

HOMEMADE APPLESAUCE

Worth the small effort.

PREPARATION

Quarter about 6 apples, leaving the skins and core, and place in a heavy pot with ¼ cup water. Set on high and then simmer, covered, for about 25 minutes until tender. Cool slightly. Put through a food mill to remove the skins and seeds. Add sugar, cinnamon, cardamom, or whatever spices you prefer to taste. Serve warm. Really good on potato pancakes (see p. 2). Makes about 1 quart.

CRANBERRY SAUCE

PREPARATION

In a large saucepan bring the orange juice and sugar to a rolling boil. Add the cranberries (if frozen, don't thaw). Bring to a boil. When the cranberry skins start popping, reduce the heat and cook, uncovered, for about 10 minutes. Remove from the heat and add the orange rind and cardamom. Cool slightly. Press through a sieve or food mill. Serve warm or cold. Tastes great as an accompaniment to poultry dishes, or as a sandwich spread with cream cheese. Makes about 3 cups.

INGREDIENTS

1 cup orange juice

1 cup sugar

1 bag fresh whole cranberries (sometimes found in the frozen food section)

Grated rind of one orange

½ teaspoon cardamom

LEMON MERINGUE CUSTARD OR CURD P

This is like lemon meringue pie without the crust. You could use lemon pudding mix or prepared lemon curd from the store, but there's no comparison to homemade.

INGREDIENTS

1 cup sugar
¼ cup cornstarch
¼ teaspoon salt
1½ cups milk
3 egg yolks, beaten
⅓ cup lemon juice
1 teaspoon lemon rind
1 teaspoon butter

LEMON CUSTARD

PREPARATION

In a double boiler combine the sugar, cornstarch, and salt. Gradually add the milk and cook over boiling water until smooth and thick, stirring constantly with a whisk. Cover and cook for 15 minutes.

Pour the egg yolks slowly into the hot mixture, stirring constantly. Cook for 5 more minutes. Add the lemon juice, lemon rind, and butter and remove from the heat. Pour into 6 ovenproof custard cups.

EASY LEMON CURD

PREPARATION

In a saucepan heat the lemon juice, sugar, and butter until the butter is melted. Add the eggs, and cook slowly until the mixture bubbles. Pour into 6 ovenproof custard cups. Cool.

INGREDIENTS

¾ cup lemon juice
2¼ cups sugar
¾ cup unsalted butter
4 eggs, beaten

MERINGUE

Think about making a meringue topping for custard when you have egg whites left over from recipes that call for egg yolks only.

PREPARATION

Preheat the oven to 350°. In a large bowl beat the egg whites until frothy. Gradually add the sugar and continue beating until stiff. Add the flavoring. Pile on top of the lemon custard or curd, making points with the tip of a knife. Bake for 10 to 15 minutes, until the peaks are slightly brown.

INGREDIENTS

3 egg whites, room temperature
6 tablespoons sugar
½ teaspoon flavoring, like vanilla or Cointreau

EGGNOG SAUCE

INGREDIENTS

1   3-ounce package
    vanilla pudding mix
2   cups milk
½   teaspoon nutmeg
½   cup Reddi Whip
2   teaspoons dark rum

PREPARATION

Cook the pudding with the milk according to package directions. Stir in the nutmeg and remove from the heat. Stir in the Reddi Whip and rum. Serve warm over pound cake. Serves about 6.

SHARTLESVILLE PUMPKIN SOUFFLÉ

PREPARATION

Preheat the oven to 450°. In a large bowl beat the pumpkin, egg yolks, sugar, salt, and spices for 5 minutes. Add the cream, butter, and whiskey and mix well. In another bowl beat the egg whites until stiff peaks form. Sprinkle the cornstarch over the egg whites and fold into the pumpkin mixture. Pour into 6 custard cups and bake for 10 minutes. Reduce the oven temperature to 350° and bake for about 30 more minutes, until the mixture is set. Top with whipped cream. Serves 6.

INGREDIENTS

1 15-ounce can pumpkin
4 eggs, separated
1 cup sugar
½ teaspoon salt
½ teaspoon cinnamon
   Dash clove, allspice, and nutmeg
⅓ cup cream
¼ cup butter, melted
¼ cup good whiskey
1 teaspoon cornstarch
   Whipped cream

INGREDIENTS

Pears (a firm pear like Bosc works well)

Apple juice

Cinnamon stick, whole cloves, cardamom, and/or ginger

Gorgonzola or feta cheese, crumbled

POACHED PEARS

PREPARATION

Pears can be firm or ripe. Peel and quarter the pears, removing the seeds. Place in a small saucepan, almost covering with apple juice. Add spices to taste. Bring to a boil, then turn down the heat and simmer, covered, for about 10 minutes. Add a little red wine before cooking if you want a richer color. Remove from the heat and let sit, covered. Serve warm or cool in a flat bowl with a little juice (remove the spices). If desired, the juice can be thickened with arrowroot or a commercial thickener (see p. xxvii). Crumble Gorgonzola or feta cheese on top.

POACHED PRUNES

PREPARATION

Soak the prunes in hot brewed tea overnight.
Drain and place the prunes in a saucepan and
cover with water. Add a few strips of lemon rind
and a little lemon juice. Bring to a boil, then
reduce the heat and simmer for about 10 minutes.
Remove the rind. Serve warm or cool with the
juice. Good covered with whipped cream.

INGREDIENTS

MANGO PURÉE

Ripe mango(es)

Fresh lime juice (2 tablespoons per mango)

Dash nutmeg

The bright orange-yellow color of mango is unique in the food world. It looks and tastes great.

PREPARATION

Peel and slice the mangoes. Purée in the blender or processor with the lime juice and nutmeg. Great as a sauce on ice cream or in yogurt or a buttermilk smoothie. Make lots and store in the fridge. Makes a great cocktail, too (see Tequila Mockingbird, p. 149). Peeled kiwi or crushed pineapple can be added for a great taste.

PAPAYA

INGREDIENTS

Makes a festive colorful breakfast first course. Papase, an enzyme in papaya as well as pineapple, also helps control excessive saliva, which can be a problem for some people with swallowing difficulties.

1 ripe papaya for 2 people

Fresh lime to taste

PREPARATION

Slice the papaya lengthwise and scoop out the seeds. Squeeze the lime juice over the fruit, or serve with a wedge of lime. Or scoop out the papaya meat for use in smoothies and sauces.

INGREDIENTS

PINEAPPLE–ORANGE BAVARIAN CRÈME

2 teaspoons unflavored gelatin

½ cup cold water

1 8-ounce can crushed pineapple

1 cup orange juice

1 teaspoon lemon juice

½ cup sugar

1 cup evaporated milk

PREPARATION

Soften the gelatin in the cold water for a few minutes. In a saucepan heat the pineapple and orange juice to boiling and add the gelatin, lemon juice, and sugar. Mix thoroughly until the gelatin is totally dissolved. Chill until partially set. Beat until light and fluffy. In a small bowl beat the evaporated milk until stiff. Fold into the gelatin. Chill until firm. Serves 8.

PEACH MELBA

PREPARATION

Skin the peaches by plunging into boiling water for 1 minute then placing immediately into cold water. The skins should peel off easily with your fingers. In a saucepan combine the sugar, water, and ¼ cup lemon juice to make the syrup. Add the peaches and poach until tender, about 5 minutes, and let cool in the syrup (omit this step if using canned peaches). Prepare the raspberry sauce by puréeing the ingredients in the processor. Pass through a strainer or food mill to remove seeds if necessary.

To serve, place a dip of vanilla ice cream in a dessert cup. Put a peach half on top with some syrup. Then drizzle raspberry sauce over all. Can be topped with whipped cream if you feel really decadent. Serves 6.

Note: You can buy raspberry sauce in specialty shops, such as Trader Joe's or Williams-Sonoma. Keep on hand when fresh raspberries are not available.

Ingredients

3 peaches, skins removed, pitted, and halved (or canned halved peaches in syrup)

Syrup:
1 cup sugar
2 cups water
¼ cup fresh lemon juice

Raspberry Sauce:
2 cups raspberries
2 teaspoons lemon juice
1 cup confectioners' sugar
Vanilla ice cream

INGREDIENTS

2 bags Oreo cookies, crushed or processed until fine
½ gallon vanilla ice cream, softened
1 17.5-ounce jar hot fudge sauce
1 12-ounce container Cool Whip

OUTRAGEOUS OREO DIRT CAKE

PREPARATION

Press half of the crushed Oreos into the bottom of a 9 x 13-inch pan. Spread the vanilla ice cream on top. Poke holes in the ice cream with a straw. Spread the hot fudge sauce (don't heat) over the ice cream layer. Spread on a layer of Cool Whip. Sprinkle the remaining half of the crushed Oreos over the Cool Whip layer. Freeze for 3 hours. Serves a crowd.

8

DRINKS

Most simple thick drinks like milk shakes and smoothies are not included here because you've probably figured out how to make them already, and most non-chew cookbooks include these. Thicker beverages are often easier to control in the mouth and while swallowing.

COFFEE

PREPARATION

Stir vanilla ice cream into hot coffee instead of
cream. The thickening agents in ice cream provide
a thicker drink. Also, the air whipped into ice
cream makes a delightful frothy drink.

MOCHA MADNESS

PREPARATION

Place all of the ingredients in the blender and process until smooth. Tastes good at room temperature or warmed in the microwave. Makes a thick drink. Serves 2.

- 1 cup freshly brewed black coffee, room temperature
- ½ banana, peeled and cut into chunks
- ⅓ cup nonfat dry milk powder
- ¼ cup ricotta cheese (a great way to use leftover ricotta)
- 1 tablespoon chocolate syrup
- ½ teaspoon vanilla extract
- 1 tablespoon sugar (or less depending on taste for sweetness)

VARIATION: MOCHA FRAPPÉ

Frappé can be a sweetened fruit juice frozen to a mushy consistency or a liqueur like crème de menthe poured over shaved ice as an after-dinner drink.

PREPARATION

Follow the above directions. With the blender motor running, add 5 to 6 ice cubes one at a time through the feeder hole in the lid until the ice is dissolved. Pour into chilled glasses.

À LA ORANGE JULIUS

INGREDIENTS

3   ounces frozen orange juice concentrate

½   cup milk (for thicker drink, use half and half)

2   cups ice

¼   cup vanilla-flavored Torani syrup, or more or less depending on preference (you've seen these syrups in upscale coffee houses, but they can also be found in the syrup section at the grocery store)

1   pasteurized egg (optional)

1   ripe banana, peeled

PREPARATION

Blend all of the ingredients in the blender for 30 seconds. Serves 2 to 3.

TROPICAL SMOOTHIE

PREPARATION

Blend all of the ingredients in the blender. Serve in glasses. Serves 4.

INGREDIENTS

1 8-ounce can crushed pineapple (use the juice)
1 cup yogurt
1 ripe banana, broken into chunks
  A few ripe strawberries, cut in half

PAPAYA–PINEAPPLE SMOOTHIE

This smoothie not only tastes great but contains papase from the papaya and pineapple juice, giving it a double dose of the enzyme that controls excess saliva.

PREPARATION

Slice the papaya in half lengthwise, scoop out the seeds, and place the scooped-out flesh in the blender. Add the other ingredients and blend until smooth. Serves 3.

INGREDIENTS

1 ripe papaya
1 5-ounce can pineapple juice
1 cup plain yogurt
  Juice of ½ lime

INGREDIENTS

1 ripe mango, peeled and meat cut from seed or 1 cup Del Monte mango in light syrup (find in a jar in the produce section)
¼ cup syrup if using fresh mango
½ cup strawberries
2 tablespoons confectioners' sugar
1 cup plain yogurt

MANGO–STRAWBERRY SMOOTHIE

PREPARATION

Mix all of the ingredients in the blender. Add a little fruit juice (apple, cranberry, or white grape) if a thinner consistency is desired. Serves 3.

KATIE DRINK

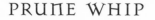

Thanks to Jo Tanzer of the ALS Association, Arizona Chapter, for this recipe.

PREPARATION

Combine all of the ingredients in the blender until smooth. Serves 4.

INGREDIENTS

½ cup cottage cheese
½ cup vanilla ice cream
1 cup gelatin (any flavor), prepared in the quick-set method but not yet refrigerated

PRUNE WHIP

PREPARATION

In the blender blend all of the ingredients on high until the skins of the prunes are the swallowing consistency you can handle. Pass through a food mill after blending to remove the skins if necessary. Serves 2.

INGREDIENTS

½ cup poached prunes, or ½ cup prune juice (pulp-free or regular)
1 cup plain yogurt
Squirt of fresh lemon
½ cup white grape juice

BRANDY ALEXANDER

INGREDIENTS

3 scoops of the best vanilla ice cream
2 ounces good brandy
1 ounce crème de cocoa
   Dash nutmeg for garnish

PREPARATION

In a blender blend the ice cream, brandy, and crème de cocoa. Serve in champagne glasses topped with nutmeg. Serves 3.

WHITE RUSSIAN

INGREDIENTS

Equal parts vodka, Kahlua, and heavy cream

PREPARATION

Pour the vodka and Kahlua over ice in a glass. Float the cream on top by pouring slowly over an upturned teaspoon.

PIÑA COLADA

INGREDIENTS

Equal parts light rum, coconut cream (find in liquor section), and fresh or canned crushed pineapple

PREPARATION

Blend the ingredients with ice in the blender.

EGGNOG

6 eggs, separated
⅓ pound sugar
½ fifth of good Kentucky bourbon
1 quart milk
1 cup heavy cream, whipped
Nutmeg for garnish

PREPARATION

In a large bowl beat the egg yolks to a froth and beat in the sugar, until the yolks are light yellow and thick. Slowly stir in the bourbon and milk. Fold in the whipped cream. In a medium bowl beat the egg whites until stiff and fold in. Sprinkle nutmeg on top of the eggnog in the punch bowl or on individual glasses. Serves a crowd.

TEQUILA MOCKINGBIRD

INGREDIENTS

½ cup mango nectar or purée (see p. 136)
2 ounces tequila
Juice of half a small lime
Splash of Triple Sec or Cointreau
Crushed ice

PREPARATION

Blend the ingredients in the blender. Serves 2.

BLOODY MARY ASPIC

½ cup vodka
Juice of ½ lime
Splash Worcestershire sauce
Dash Tabasco
½ teaspoon horseradish
1 packet unflavored gelatin
12 ounces tomato juice, heated

PREPARATION

In a 2-cup measuring cup, combine the vodka, lime juice, Worcestershire, Tabasco, and horseradish. Sprinkle the gelatin on top and let stand a minute or two. Pour in the hot tomato juice and stir until dissolved, about 2 minutes. Pour into tiny specialty cups and refrigerate until firm, about 2 hours. Serves about 6 as an appetizer.

JELL-O SHOOTERS

1 3-ounce package lime gelatin
½ cup vodka

PREPARATION

Prepare the gelatin using the speed-set method, replacing ½ cup cold water with the vodka. Pour into a square pan (or individual small paper cups) and refrigerate for about 2 hours, until firm. Cut into cubes and pop into mouth or squeeze into mouth from paper cup. This is a real conversation piece at a party. Serves about 8.

CHAGALL'S PURPLE COW

PREPARATION

Blend all ingredients in the blender. Serves 2.

INGREDIENTS

2 scoops vanilla ice cream

½ cup grape juice

¼ cup vodka

Appendix

Puréed Foods

FOODS FOR KIDS

Menus for Special Occasions

Appetizers:

Bangkok Butternut Squash Soup, 85
Blended Salad, 96
Brie Soup, 72
Crab Louise, 98

Leslie's Zucchini Bisque, 77
Salmon Pâté, 32
Shrimp Salad, 99
Yin Yang Soup, 70–71

Entrées and Sides:

Braised Lamb and Eggplant Provençale (p. 48) with Blended Salad (p. 96)
Grilled Filet Mignon and Portobello Mushrooms (p. 38) with Pesto Mashed Potatoes (p. 8)
Kentucky-Style Stewed Chicken and Dumplings (p. 45) with Cranberry Sauce (p. 129), Coleslaw (p. 97), and Claudia's Southwestern Yams (p. 10) (and if you add Shartlesville Pumpkin

Soufflé [p. 133], this menu works well for Thanksgiving dinner)
Mushroom Crêpes and Goat Cheese Sauce (p. 28–29) with Glazed Carrots (p. 26)
Vanessa's Green Chile Chicken Enchiladas (p. 42) with Guacamole (p. 116) and Sautéed Spinach (p. 14)

Desserts:

Black Russian Bundt Cake, 127
Chocolate Cake Pudding with Bourbon Sauce, 125

Poached Pears with Crumbled Gorgonzola Cheese, 134

Index

About the Author

Elayne Achilles, who has won various cooking competitions, is a professor at Arizona State University. She has written for numerous professional publications and has served as an editor for the *Music Educators Journal* and other similar journals. She lives in Phoenix, Arizona.